Personalized Psychiatry

Ives Cavalcante Passos • Benson Mwangi
Flávio Kapczinski
Editors

Personalized Psychiatry

Big Data Analytics in Mental Health

Springer

Editors
Ives Cavalcante Passos
Laboratory of Molecular Psychiatry
Hospital de Clinicas de Porto Alegre
Porto Alegre, Brazil

Programa de Pós-Graduação em Psiquiatria e Ciências do Comportamento
Universidade Federal do Rio Grande do Sul
Porto Alegre, Brazil

Flávio Kapczinski
Department of Psychiatry and Behavioural Neurosciences
McMaster University
Hamilton, ON, Canada

Benson Mwangi
UT Center of Excellence on Mood Disorders
Department of Psychiatry and Behavioral Sciences
The University of Texas Health Science Center at Houston
McGovern Medical School
Houston, TX, USA

ISBN 978-3-030-03552-5 ISBN 978-3-030-03553-2 (eBook)
https://doi.org/10.1007/978-3-030-03553-2

Library of Congress Control Number: 2018968426

This Springer imprint is published by the registered company Springer Nature Switzerland AG.
The registered company address is: Gewerbestrasse 11, 6330 Cham, Switzerland

Foreword

Big Data Is Watching You

These are exciting times in the history of psychiatry for a number of reasons. First and foremost, with mapping of the brain and functioning of various parts, it is getting closer to our understanding of cognitions and emotions. Both researchers and clinicians are beginning to understand the role of genome and psychopharmacogenomics is beginning to guide prescription patterns of psychiatric diseases. Trials are under way to indicate which of our patients are fast metabolisers and which are slow metabolisers so that targeted doses of medication can be used in gaining the optimum effect. At one level, psychiatry has always been personalised because the patients sitting in front of us even with similar symptoms have very different responses to therapeutic interactions. Who will respond to which treatment needs big data. With an increase in the use of social media, personal apps for managing some distress and symptoms, the importance of data and information cannot be underestimated. One of the earliest interventions in psychiatry was psychoanalysis analysing the individual to make sense of their experiences and development. The practice of psychiatry has moved on from analysis by human beings to analysis of data by machines which has its advantages and disadvantages.

Various authors in this volume remind us that human beings have always been interested in big data. Data is collected on individuals from birth to death. Some countries have major data sets on each citizen creating thousands of variables which can enable us to make sense of individual experiences in the context of larger social structures be they health or social care.

Predictive psychiatry is an exciting new field where using large data sets may allow us to predict responses and outcomes. Machines such as smartphones and computers are an integral part of human functioning and human lives. Designed algorithms tell us that if we liked a particular book or song, we are likely to prefer book B or song B. These algorithms can be helpful. In the recent WPA-Lancet Psychiatry Commission on the Future of Psychiatry (Bhugra et al. 2017), one of the recommendations was that psychiatrists need to be up-to-date in the evolving digital world bearing in mind the potential risks of commercialised unproven treatments and interventions. However, as long as wider collaboration between stakeholders is maintained, it should be possible to reap the rewards of digital psychiatry, and this volume provides an excellent example of that. Widely used digital tools and their ability to collect huge data sets or deliver services related to mental and physical health are only now beginning to be realised. The reality of digital psychiatry is certainly not without its challenges, and authors in this volume tackle these head-on.

In clinical psychiatry, there has been a long tradition of analysing history and the patient in the context of their development, and at one level, it appears frightening and scary that machines can do this for our decisions be they clinical or nonclinical. In the past 2 decades, computers, smartphones, and social media algorithms have both enriched our lives and also produced a feeling of concern as to where this might lead. These interactions are based on algorithms which are also used in clinical decision-making relying on evidence based more so in some medical specialities rather than others. Digital psychiatry can contribute a tremendous amount of support to clinicians especially when patients and their doctors live miles apart. There are already innovative practices using e-mental health and tele-mental health practices in many parts of the world.

The access to new technologies may well vary across countries, but with an increased use of smartphones around the world means that levels of physical activities, pulse rates and blood pressure can be easily measured and monitored. New technologies may enable mental health and physical health to be integrated more readily than has been the case so far. As is clear from contributions to this unique and excellent volume, the data sets generated from the use of machines such as smartphones and laptops can help us make sense of wellbeing of individuals. Thus, close collaboration between data scientists and psychiatrists as well as other mental health professionals is critical to help develop algorithms for future understanding of personalised clinical practice. This volume offers a unique viewpoint and insight on the journey in scientific development of psychiatry.

Big data on the one hand comprises of velocity, volume, and variety which are readily visible in our use of smartphones. As several authors in this volume remind us, the data can be stored, and yet rapid access to billions of data sets with capacity increases on a daily basis. As is strongly emphasised in this volume, big data for psychiatry is unlike any other. Data related to investigations including brain scans and other neuroimaging studies can also contribute to big data. Big data can also help collect large sets of phenotypes to facilitate our understanding of biological causes of mental illnesses and enable suitable personalised interventions. These data sets can facilitate development of individualised nosology of psychiatric disorders perhaps moving away from one-size-fits-all phenomenology.

Of course, there are critical issues related to confidentiality, probity, and security in data collection and data management of clinical matters. On the other hand, patients do not fit into tight categories of the machine-generated algorithms. Such information should be seen as supplementary sources of information, e.g. ascertaining physical activities and not only information while reaching a clinical diagnosis or planning therapeutic interventions. However, it is also important that clinicians are taught and trained how to use these resources properly and appropriately.

The editors and authors in this splendid volume are to be congratulated for their vision and pioneering spirit which hopefully will lead to better, individualised, and focused care of patients with psychiatric problems.

Reference

Bhugra D, Tasman A, Pathare S, et al (2017) The WPA-lancet commission on the future of psychiatry. Lancet Psychiatry 4:775–818

Emeritus Professor, Mental Health and Cultural Diversity
IoPPN, Kings College, London, UK
Dinesh Bhugra

Preface

This book was written to address the emerging need to deal with the explosion of information available about individual behaviours and choices. Importantly, we believe that there are still untapped opportunities to transform such information into intelligence that would enable personalised care in mental health.

Our unprecedented ability to gain knowledge about each individual will be paramount in allowing us to implement personalised care in mental health. Ground-breaking discoveries and changes at the population level will involve data integration enabling a person-centred approach. Big data tools will be needed to assess the phenome, genome, and exposome of patients. That will include data from imaging, insurance, pharmacy, social media, as well as *-omics* data (genomics, proteomics, and metabolomics). Briefly, big data are characterised by high volume, high velocity, and variety. We believe therefore that attention has to shift to new analytical tools from the field of machine learning and artificial intelligence that will be critical for anyone practicing medicine, psychiatry, and behavioural sciences in the twenty-first century.

Integration of data from multiple levels can be translated into clinical practice by both the generation of homogeneous groups of patients and the use of calculators to accurately predict outcomes at an individual level. That will facilitate important clinical decisions. An inventive approach to big data analytics in mental health will be needed to translate data from large and complex datasets into the care of consumers. That will transform predictions and information into a greater understanding of risk assessment and better mental health care.

Personalised interventions will be the outcome of the development of this field. Innovative methods for risk assessment will allow the development of personalised interventions at the level of prevention, treatment, and rehabilitation. A creative approach to big data analytics in mental health will be crucial in promoting, generating, and testing new interventions for mental health problems. Big data analytics will be at the core of the next level of innovation in mental health care. Thus, our vision for the future is a world in which mental health professionals will have the tools to deal with multilevel information that will provide patients and caregivers with the intelligence needed to enable better care.

This book will benefit clinicians, practitioners, and scientists in the fields of psychiatry, psychology, and behavioural sciences and ultimately patients with mental illness. We also intend to reach graduate and undergraduate students in these fields. Our main aims are (1) to empower researchers with a different way to conceptualise studies in mental health by using big data analytics approaches; (2) to provide clinicians with a broad perspective about how clinical decisions such as treatment options, preventive strategies, and prognosis orientations will be transformed by big data approaches; (3) to provide a unique opportunity to showcase innovative solutions tackling complex problems in mental health using big data and machine learning; and (4) to discuss challenges in terms of what data could be used without jeopardising individual privacy and freedom.

This volume has a total of nine chapters, which are structured as follows: Chapter 1 introduces the concepts of big data and machine learning and also provides a historical perspective of how big data analytics meet health sciences. Chapter 2 explores the challenges and limitations of machine learning—the most important technique to analyse big data. Chapter 3 provides a clinical perspective on big data in mental health. Chapters 4 and 5 present the state of art of tools to predict treatment response and suicide, respectively. Chapter 6 explores the emerging shifts in neuroimaging data analysis, while Chapter 7 discusses methods, such as unsupervised machine learning, for deconstructing diagnosis in mental health. Chapter 8 describes how to integrate data from multiple biological layers to build multimodal signatures. Lastly, Chapter 9 addresses ethics in the era of big data.

Contributors of this book are true leaders of this emerging field and are fostering a revolution from the existing evidence medicine and traditional average group-level studies to the current personalised care scenario. In this new paradigm, large and complex datasets will be digested into calculators and predictive tools. These will provide clinicians with real-time intelligence that will guide personalised care in mental health.

Porto Alegre, RS, Brazil — Ives Cavalcante Passos
Houston, TX, USA — Benson Mwangi
Hamilton, ON, Canada — Flávio Kapczinski

Contents

Contributors

Pedro Ballester School of Technology, Pontifícia Universidade Católica do Rio Grande do Sul, Porto Alegre, Brazil

Samantha L. Bernecker Department of Psychology, Harvard University, Cambridge, MA, USA

Robert M. Bossarte Departments of Behavioral Medicine and Psychiatry, West Virginia University School of Medicine, Morgantown, WV, USA

U.S. Department of Veterans Affairs Center of Excellence for Suicide Prevention, Canandaigua, NY, USA

Danilo Bzdok Department of Psychiatry and Psychotherapy, RWTH Aachen University, Aachen, Germany

Jülich Aachen Research Alliance (JARA)—Translational Brain Medicine, Aachen, Germany

Parietal Team, INRIA, Gif-sur-Yvette, France

Bo Cao Department of Psychiatry, Faculty of Medicine & Dentistry, University of Alberta, Edmonton, AB, Canada

Richard Dinga Department of Psychiatry, Amsterdam Neuroscience and Amsterdam Public Health Research Institute, VU University Medical Center, Amsterdam, The Netherlands

Flávio Kapczinski Department of Psychiatry and Behavioural Neurosciences, McMaster University, Hamilton, ON, Canada

Siegfried Kasper Medical University of Vienna, Department for Psychiatry and Psychotherapy, Vienna, Austria

Alexander Kautzky Medical University of Vienna, Department for Psychiatry and Psychotherapy, Vienna, Austria

Matcheri Keshavan Department of Psychiatry, Beth Israel Deaconess Medical Center, Harvard Medical School, Boston, MA, USA

Ronald C. Kessler Department of Health Care Policy, Harvard Medical School, Boston, MA, USA

Rupert Lanzenberger Medical University of Vienna, Department for Psychiatry and Psychotherapy, Vienna, Austria

Diego Librenza-Garcia Department of Psychiatry and Behavioural Neurosciences, McMaster University, Mood Disorders Program, Hamilton, ON, Canada

Graduation Program in Psychiatry and Department of Psychiatry, Federal University of Rio Grande do Sul (UFRGS), Porto Alegre, Brazil

Martin Lindquist Department of Biostatistics, Johns Hopkins University, Baltimore, MD, USA

Alex R. Luedtke Vaccine and Infectious Disease Division, Fred Hutchinson Cancer Research Center, Seattle, WA, USA

Andre F. Marquand Donders Centre for Cognitive Neuroimaging, Donders Institute for Brain, Cognition and Behaviour, Radboud University, Nijmegen, The Netherlands

Department of Cognitive Neuroscience, Radboud University Medical Centre, Nijmegen, The Netherlands

Department of Neuroimaging, Centre for Neuroimaging Sciences, Institute of Psychiatry, King's College London, London, UK

John F. McCarthy Serious Mental Illness Treatment Resource and Evaluation Center, Office of Mental Health Operations, VA Center for Clinical Management Research, Ann Arbor, MI, USA

Benson Mwangi UT Center of Excellence on Mood Disorders, Department of Psychiatry and Behavioral Sciences, The University of Texas Health Science Center at Houston, McGovern Medical School, Houston, TX, USA

Nikan Namiri Department of Bioengineering, University of California Los Angeles, Los Angeles, CA, USA

Matthew K. Nock Department of Psychology, Harvard University, Cambridge, MA, USA

Ives Cavalcante Passos Laboratory of Molecular Psychiatry, Hospital de Clinicas de Porto Alegre, Porto Alegre, Brazil

Programa de Pós-Graduação em Psiquiatria e Ciências do Comportamento, Universidade Federal do Rio Grande do Sul, Porto Alegre, Brazil

Maria V. Petukhova Department of Health Care Policy, Harvard Medical School, Boston, MA, USA

Wilfred R. Pigeon Departments of Behavioral Medicine and Psychiatry, West Virginia University School of Medicine, Morgantown, WV, USA

U.S. Department of Veterans Affairs Center of Excellence for Suicide Prevention, Canandaigua, NY, USA

Jairo Vinícius Pinto Laboratory of Molecular Psychiatry, Hospital de Clinicas de Porto Alegre, Porto Alegre, Brazil

Programa de Pós-Graduação em Psiquiatria e Ciências do Comportamento, Universidade Federal do Rio Grande do Sul, Porto Alegre, Brazil

Sergey M. Plis The Mind Research Network, Albuquerque, NM, USA

Jim Reilly Department of Electrical and Computer Engineering, McMaster University, Hamilton, ON, Canada

Ekaterina Sadikova Department of Health Care Policy, Harvard Medical School, Boston, MA, USA

Marc-Andre Schulz Department of Psychiatry and Psychotherapy, RWTH Aachen University, Aachen, Germany

Rogers F. Silva The Mind Research Network, Albuquerque, NM, USA

John Torous Division of Digital Psychiatry, Beth Israel Deaconess Medical Center, Harvard Medical School, Boston, MA, USA

Department of Psychiatry, Beth Israel Deaconess Medical Center, Harvard Medical School, Boston, MA, USA

Tyler J. VanderWeele Department of Biostatistics, Harvard T.H. Chan School of Public Health, Boston, MA, USA

Department of Epidemiology, Harvard T.H. Chan School of Public Health, Boston, MA, USA

Thomas Wolfers Donders Centre for Cognitive Neuroimaging, Donders Institute for Brain, Cognition and Behaviour, Radboud University, Nijmegen, The Netherlands

Department of Human Genetics, Radboud University Medical Centre, Nijmegen, The Netherlands

Alan M. Zaslavsky Department of Health Care Policy, Harvard Medical School, Boston, MA, USA

Kelly L. Zuromski Department of Psychology, Harvard University, Cambridge, MA, USA

Big Data and Machine Learning Meet the Health Sciences

1

Ives Cavalcante Passos, Pedro Ballester, Jairo Vinícius Pinto, Benson Mwangi, and Flávio Kapczinski

Humanity was built upon large amounts of data recorded in many forms. From birth, the human being is flooded with information from multiple sources. Early in life these sources emanated from our bodies and from the small environment that surrounded us. Through our sensory nervous system we gathered information from the world around us and stored this in our brains. Over the next years of our lives, we learned to interpret other forms of information and more complex data. Without this process of interpretation and storage of large amounts of information, the brain and our humanity could not become fully developed. So, it can be sensibly concluded that human history is the story of learning and interpreting information, and storing and using this information to modify our environment, to solve problems and to improve our lives.

I. C. Passos (✉) · J. V. Pinto
Laboratory of Molecular Psychiatry, Hospital de Clinicas de Porto Alegre, Porto Alegre, Brazil

Programa de Pós-Graduação em Psiquiatria e Ciências do Comportamento, Universidade Federal do Rio Grande do Sul, Porto Alegre, Brazil
e-mail: ivescp1@gmail.com; jairovinicius@msn.com

P. Ballester
School of Technology, Pontifícia Universidade Católica do Rio Grande do Sul, Porto Alegre, Brazil
e-mail: pedballester@gmail.com

B. Mwangi
UT Center of Excellence on Mood Disorders, Department of Psychiatry and Behavioral Sciences, The University of Texas Health Science Center at Houston, McGovern Medical School, Houston, TX, USA
e-mail: benson.mwangi@gmail.com

F. Kapczinski
Department of Psychiatry and Behavioural Neurosciences, McMaster University, Hamilton, ON, Canada
e-mail: flavio.kapczinski@gmail.com

I. C. Passos et al., *Personalized Psychiatry*,
https://doi.org/10.1007/978-3-030-03553-2_1

Big data is a broad term used to denote volumes of large and complex measurements, as well as the velocity at which data is created. Another crucial characteristic of big data is the variety of levels at which data is created, from the molecular level, including genomics, proteomics and metabolomics, to clinical, sociodemographic, administrative, environmental, and even social media information (Passos et al. 2016). It could be said that we are living the "big data era"; however, humanity has always been surrounded by variable amounts of information. So, what differentiates current times from the past? Nowadays, we can collect and store large amounts of data that cannot be interpreted by humans without using powerful computational techniques. Big data therefore also reflects the core of a new world that has emerged quickly, a world with various types of technologies related to data storage, data processing and its use, and the potential to improve our society in many positive ways (Klous and Wielaard 2016).

The search of patterns in the data to enable relevant conclusions is an important part of big data. A range of techniques in computer algorithms used to identify patterns of interaction among variables has been developed over the last few decades and grouped under the name of machine learning, also known as pattern recognition, to interpret and make data-driven decisions using big datasets. Machine learning comes from the artificial intelligence field and uses mathematical functions to give computer systems the ability to "learn" from experiences and make predictions on data, without being explicitly programmed (Mitchell and Tom 1997). The engineer Arthur Samuel developed one of the first programs based on machine learning techniques in 1956. He wanted to create a computer that could beat him at checkers and had the computer playing against itself thousands of times in order to learn. The Samuel Checkers-playing Program was one of the world's first successful self-learning programs, and as such is a very early demonstration of the fundamental concept of machine learning—Samuel actually coined the term "machine learning" in 1959. In 1962, his program was able to beat Robert Nealey, a Connecticut state champion of checkers, in an historic event.

By 1997, however, when a computer called Deep Blue defeated Garry Kasparov, the world chess champion, for the first time, machine learning methods were somewhat forgotten. At that time, traditional methods, usually called Good Old-Fashioned Artificial Intelligence (GOFAI), were paving the way for artificial intelligence advances. GOFAI limitations and its need for human expertise on modelling problems were soon discovered, and, to this date, GOFAI methods are still unable to beat humans at more complex games. This has brought machine learning back to the core of artificial intelligence research. Its application for board games culminated in 2017, when AlphaGO Zero, a self-taught machine powered by a novel field of machine learning called Deep Learning, beat the world champion of Go, an ancient Chinese board game (Silver et al. 2017). Go is claimed to be one of the world's most complex games due to its combinatorial explosion at every move. In that scenario, the machine was able to learn Go only by playing with itself numerous times and identifying which moves led to a higher win rate.

Nowadays, the use of machine learning has greatly increased and goes far beyond the gaming tables. A number of activities in our daily routines are facilitated by these techniques. Perhaps machine learning's first big success in commercial use was Google, a search engine that uses these techniques to organize world information. Similarly, machine learning is used by Facebook to suggest friends and by Netflix to suggest movies and TV shows. Another interesting invention that takes advantage of machine learning is predictive policing, named as one of the 50 best inventions of 2011 (TIME 2011). This breakthrough refers to the use of machine learning techniques in law enforcement to identify potential criminal activity. In the United States, police departments in Arizona, California, Illinois, South Carolina, Tennessee, and Washington have implemented the practice of predictive policing. The aim is to develop models for predicting crimes, offenders, and victims of crime, and guide utilization of scarce policing resources.

How do computers or machines actually learn? Generally, machines receive data from a certain sensor following an unknown distribution and fit mathematical functions that best explain the data. Noteworthy are some algorithms that allow the modelling of any function, called universal function approximators, thus removing the need for humans to try different equations or distributions (as is common in traditional statistical analysis). The process of fitting, mostly called training, is usually performed in three different ways, which diverge mainly on whether and how an expected outcome variable is presented. In the first scenario, called unsupervised learning, the machine usually aims at finding the best way to group data by similarity with no additional knowledge about the task (Bishop 2006). In supervised learning, machines receive data with the outcome. The function is then modelled to best predict the outcome based on the predictors (Bishop 2006). Those two paradigms are frequently mixed, defining what is called semi-supervised learning, a paradigm that leverages knowledge from a task using examples both with and without annotated outcome. Lastly, reinforcement learning is a training paradigm analogous to animal training. There is no fixed outcome variable; here the machine, called an agent because of its ability to interact with the environment, is "rewarded" or "punished" every time it performs the task appropriately, with the aim of maximizing the total reward received (Sutton and Barto 1998). Reinforcement learning mirrors the well-known principle of operant conditioning in psychology where a behavior is modified through positive reinforcements or rewards and punishments. Supervised and unsupervised learning are the most frequent paradigms in the health sciences literature.

How is a study with machine learning designed? For complex questions, such as those faced in mental health and behavior sciences, big datasets are generally needed. In supervised learning, the algorithm analyzes a "training" dataset drawn from the original dataset to establish candidate models able to distinguish individual subjects across levels of a specific outcome (Fig. 1.1). Model tuning and feature reductions routines could be implemented to improve model performance (fully discussed in Chap. 2). The best model is then applied to a new dataset, and its performance can be measured in this new scenario. As a result, the algorithm can predict the probability of an outcome at an individual level. This prediction may be, for example, the likelihood of a Netflix client liking a movie or the probability of a patient developing heart disease. In Chap. 7 we address how unsupervised learning studies are implemented.

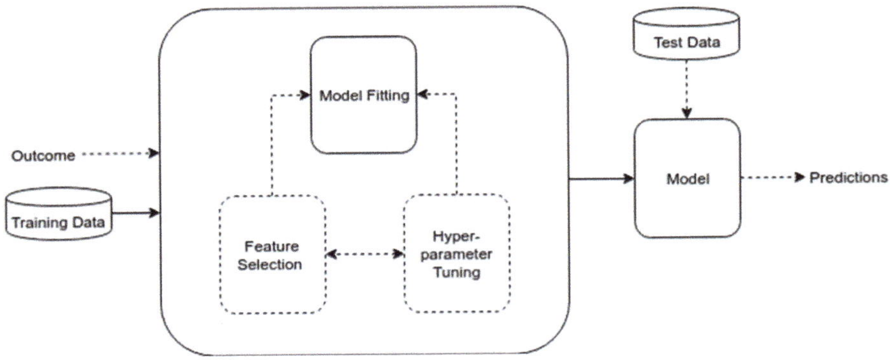

Fig. 1.1 A standard machine learning training protocol. The outcome and test data may be neither available nor applicable to the desired task

Big data analytics with the use of machine learning techniques are gaining traction in health sciences and might provide predictive models for both clinical practice and public health systems. Chapter 3 will provide a complete clinical perspective of how big data and machine learning techniques will help to improve care in mental disorders. However, before exploring their impact on mental health care, we will offer a concise historical overview of some important events in health sciences through the lens of epidemiology. Mervyn Susser and Ezra Susser wrote about three eras in epidemiology covering the period following the Industrial Revolution (Susser and Susser 1996). Each era introduced new ways of thinking about the causes of illnesses in the face of particular problems, such as the cholera outbreak in London or the increasing rates of chronic noncommunicable diseases after World War II. *More importantly, each era and its problems challenged researchers to find and to develop new analytical methods to find causes and improve health.* This knowledge is important to understand why big data and machine learning have recently become promising methods to define, predict, and treat illnesses, and how they can transform the way we conceptualize care in medicine. As Mervyn Susser and Ezra Susser stated in their work "to look forward, we do well to look backward for guidance."

1.1 Eras of Epidemiology: Paradigms and Analytical Approach

The miasma theory was the prevailing paradigm to explain the etiopathogenesis of diseases such as cholera in the nineteenth century. It stated that the etiology of some diseases was related to a noxious vapor that arose from decaying organic matter such as sewage. In 1854, John Snow challenged this theory during a cholera outbreak in Soho, London. By talking to victims or their families, he detected the source of the outbreak in London as the public water pump located at Broad Street (now Broadwick Street). His studies of the pattern of the disease established that cholera

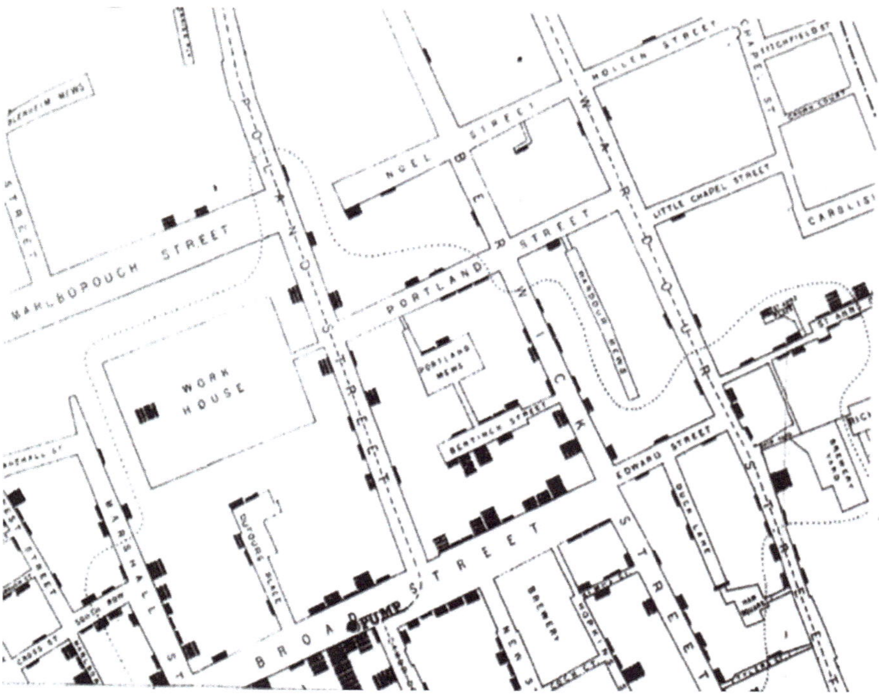

Fig. 1.2 John Snow's dot map showed the association between cases of cholera and proximity to the Broad Street pump

was transmitted by the water supply, and convinced the local authorities to disable the water pump. John Snow later utilized a dot map to depicits the cluster of cholera cases close to the pump (Fig. 1.2). It is regarded as one of the founding events in the science of epidemiology and he is renowned for being one of the fathers of modern epidemiology.

John Snow's work and actions have been commonly credited for ending the cholera outbreak. It is noteworthy that he discovered that a profitable water supply was the primary mode of cholera transmission well before the discovery of the vibrio cholera bacterium by collecting data and interpreting its pattern in the Soho area. This event illustrates the sanitary era, which was marked by the sanitary statistics collected as evidence at the societal level and related to overall morbidity and mortality data. This analytical approach guided the interventions for cleaner urban water supplies and sewage systems. The following excerpt illustrates John Snow's methods in his search for a cause of the cholera outbreak (Snow 1854, pp. 321–322).

> I requested permission, therefore, to take a list at the General Register Office of the deaths from cholera registered during the week ending September 2, in the sub-districts of Golden-square, Berwick-street, and St. Ann's, Soho. Eighty-nine deaths from cholera were registered during the week, in the three sub-districts. Of these, only six occurred in the four first days of the week, four occurred on Thursday, the 31st ult., and the remaining

> seventy-nine on Friday and Saturday. I considered, therefore, that the outbreak commenced on the Thursday; and I made an inquiry, in detail, respecting the eighty-three deaths registered as having taken place during the last three days of the week. On proceeding to the spot, I found that nearly all the deaths had taken place within a short distance of the pump. There were only ten deaths in houses situated decidedly nearer to another street pump. In five of these cases the families of the deceased persons informed me that they always sent to the pump in Broad-street, as they preferred the water to that of the pumps which were nearer. In three other cases the deceased were children who went to school near the pump in Broad-street. Two of them were known to drink the water, and the parents of the third think it probable that it did so. The other two deaths, beyond the district which this pump supplies, represent only the amount of mortality from cholera that was occurring before the eruption took place. With regard to the deaths occurring in the locality belonging to the pump, there were 61 instances in which I was informed that the deceased persons used to drink the pump water from Broad-street, either constantly or occasionally. In six instances I could get no information, owing to the death or departure of every one connected with the deceased individuals; and in six cases I was informed that the deceased persons did not drink the pump water before their illness.
>
> The result of this inquiry, then, is, that there has been no particular outbreak or prevalence of cholera in this part of London except among the persons who were in the habit of drinking the water of the above-mentioned pump-well.

In 1883, Robert Koch finally isolated the comma bacillus in pure culture and explained its mode of transmission, solving an enigma that had lasted for centuries (Lippi and Gotuzzo 2014). This discovery and the works of Louis Pasteur and Jakob Henle opened up new avenues of innovation and brought health sciences into the infectious disease era at the turn of the century. The research and epidemiology in medicine therefore underwent a dramatic paradigm shift fostered by the new science of microbiology, which had produced definitive evidence of a causative relationship between microbes and human disease. Instead of focusing on societal-level causes and sanitary statistics, methods in this era included the development of bacteriology laboratories, culture from disease sites, and microbe isolation. The goal was to detect the "*sufficient*" and "*necessary*" cause of a disease. These concepts were embodied in the famous Henle-Koch postulates for establishing an infectious agent as a cause of disease. The postulates require that the causative agent be absent in individuals without the disease and present in all individuals with the disease. This progress in the field of microbiology also advanced the fields of drug interventions and vaccinations. For instance, the discovery of the spirochete that causes syphilis was followed by the development of Salvarsan 606, the first drug agent against an infectious disease, so named because it took 606 experiments to find the effective compound (Susser 2006).

After World War II, noncommunicable chronic diseases, such as cardiovascular diseases, cancer, chronic respiratory diseases, and diabetes, were increasing at an alarming rate while infectious diseases were declining in developed countries. In this context, the singular notion of necessary and sufficient causes was replaced by the concept of risk factors, that is, a combination of factors from multiple biological levels causes the disease, and each factor increases the probability of disease in an individual (Susser 2006). In this sense, we assume that diseases are produced by multiple interacting causes and that the same disease may be caused through different, sometimes unknown, pathways. Therefore, methods for identifying risk factors, such as case–control and cohort designs, were developed. This was the risk factor era, which began after World War II and persists to this day. At the dawn of this era, mental disorders were counted among the important chronic diseases to be investigated. One of the earliest and most influential works was Lee Robin's investigation of the relationship between childhood behavior problems and adult antisocial behavior by following up children after a period of 30 years (Robins 1966). We can also highlight the studies conducted by Avalom Caspi, which formed the pillars of the gene–environment model. Caspi and colleagues showed that a functional polymorphism in the gene encoding the enzyme monoamine oxidase A (MAO-A) moderated the effect of maltreatment. Children who suffered abuse and who presented a genotype that conferred low levels of MAO-A expression were more likely to develop antisocial problems while those who exhibited high levels of this enzyme were less likely to demonstrate antisocial behavior (Caspi et al. 2002). However, the causal chain of chronic diseases, including mental disorders, is much more complex than the linear gene–environment interactions. This field needs powerful multivariate techniques that are able to model complex interactions, commonly nonlinear associations, among factors from multiple biological levels in order to not only define and treat these chronic diseases but also to predict them and to orient their prognosis—*which is why big data and machine learning techniques meet health science.*

Each prior era focused on a specific biological level; however, multilevel thinkers are now in evidence. Compared with traditional statistical methods that provide primarily average group-level results, machine learning algorithms allow predictions and stratification of clinical outcomes at the level of an individual subject. Machine learning can also yield better relationship estimations between multivariate data. By theoretically being able to model any function, machines can find complex nonlinear patterns relating predictors to their expected outcome (Obermeyer and Emanuel 2016). Traditional statistical analysis, however, usually fails to find models with nonlinearities and even in some more optimistic scenarios, still cannot cope with high-degree polynomial patterns.

Nowadays, all major psychiatric disorders have been studied with machine learning techniques, including schizophrenia, bipolar disorder, major depressive disorder, post-traumatic stress disorder, attention deficit hyperactivity disorder, and substance use disorders. Moreover, the studies have included analysis of different biological levels as predictors, including socio-demographics and clinical variables (Kessler et al. 2014), peripheral biomarkers (Pinto et al. 2017), neuroimaging (Mwangi et al. 2016; Wu et al. 2017; Librenza-Garcia et al. 2017; Sartori et al. 2018), and neuropsychological tests (Wu et al. 2016). Despite their innovative approach, some of these studies included only small sample sizes, had cross-section designs, were still pilot studies, and lacked external validation. Chapter 2 will explore these limitations further and discuss the obstacles that are faced.

1.2 The Dawn of the Intelligent Therapeutic Interventions

Chapter 4 will provide a synthesis of studies that used big data and machine learning techniques to select treatment intervention. Therein, we will conceptualize how big data and machine learning may help evidence-based medicine toward personalized care.

Prediction of treatment response at an individual patient level remains an elusive goal for some chronic illnesses, including mental disorders. For instance, selecting an antipsychotic medication for schizophrenia remains a trial-and-error process, with no specific biomarkers to lend decision support. Randomized clinical trials and meta-analyses, the pillars of evidence-based medicine, have helped us to identify effective treatments for specific disorders by leveraging traditional statistical methods (Evidence-Based Medicine Working Group 1992). Traditional statistical methods as mentioned above primarily provide average group-level results within a population. On the one hand, this approach allows us to make broad generalizations about a specific population in regard to a specific drug. On the other hand, it fails to detect nuances related to an individual subject, and significant results may not represent a real benefit for some (Greenhalgh et al. 2014). Indeed, subjects included in clinical trials frequently do not reflect patients from real-world clinical scenarios. In the latter, patients have different multimorbidity profiles, severity of symptoms, degree of functional impairment, and even cultural backgrounds compared to the former—and all these factors may play a role in treatment response. Consequently, big data and machine learning guided intervention trials may help evidence-based medicine by using these nuances to make predictions of treatment response (and side effects) at an individual level. It is important to note that both clinical practitioners and machine learning algorithms seek to accumulate knowledge from previous patients and translate it to each new patient's case.

Several studies have attempted to find a single biomarker that can predict those patients who are likely to respond to a specific medication but results have not been consistently replicated. Several features or predictors ranging from genetics, molecular or neuroanatomical levels, to population, demographic and social levels may be associated with better outcomes of one treatment as opposed to another. Markedly, they may have little predictive value on their own but, when combined, they lead to improved predictive utility. For instance, Chekroud and colleagues built a multimodal machine learning tool composed of clinical and demographic data to predict treatment response to antidepressants (Chekroud et al. 2016). This tool was subsequently validated using an external sample. Additionally, Cao and colleagues reported a clinical tool able to predict response to risperidone treatment in first-episode drug-naive schizophrenia patients with a balanced accuracy of 82.5% (Cao et al. 2018) by using powerful machine learning techniques to analyze multivariate data from resting-state functional magnetic resonance imaging (fMRI). Models like these can be displayed as a user-friendly calculator, and incorporated into clinical workflows including electronic medical records. In the case where the calculator predicts that a patient is unlikely to respond to a specific medication, the clinician can consider alternative medications and the patients will not endure prolonged periods of "trial-and-error" in search of the right treatment and the burden associated with this process. Additionally, another unexplored outcome is the prediction of side effects, such as hyperprolactinemia in patients taking risperidone, which could also assist in treatment selection.

A focus on individuals, rather than group-level averages, by using big data and machine learning models that could leverage each person's unique biological profile to improve selection of treatment, may bring personalized care to psychiatry. This is important since over the past decade the field has not developed more efficient drugs to treat schizophrenia, for instance. A network meta-analysis published in 2013 showed that the new antipsychotic drugs at that time, such as asenapine, iloperidone, and lurasidone, had the worst efficacy in treating psychosis (Leucht et al. 2013). However, there are some obstacles to be overcome before models like those published by Chekroud and Cao are translated into actual clinical applications: (1) the cost related to some methods, such as fMRI, is still prohibitive; and (2) it is unclear at this stage whether the proposed models are broadly representative.

1.3 Devices and Patient Empowerment

Another interesting angle to the impact of big data and machine learning on health science is the way in which data is collected and stored. The development of devices to assess data (sometimes real-time streaming data throughout a patient's daily activities), to analyze the data, and to give clinical insights not only for clinicians but also for patients, will also redefine care in health sciences. During World War II, the English mathematician Alan Turing studied cryptoanalysis to crack the intercepted German Enigma code, which was a crucial step in enabling the Allies to defeat the Nazis. The theory behind the machine that would break the Enigma code dates back to 1936, and Alan Turing's seminal paper (Turing 1937). Alongside building the first computational model, Alan Turing questioned whether those machines could 1 day actually think, and proposed that machines should be expected to compete with humans in intellectual tasks in years to come (Turing 1950). Alan Turing is considered to be the father of computer science and artificial intelligence.

Much like Turing's prediction, machines are competing with, and in some cases surpassing, human being's abilities in intellectual tasks. A successful example of the use of devices based on machine learning techniques comes from ophthalmology (Ting et al. 2017). In 2018, The U.S. Food and Drug Administration (FDA) approved the first medical device that uses machine learning techniques to detect diabetic retinopathy. The director of the Division of Ophthalmic, and Ear, Nose and Throat Devices at the FDA's Center for Devices and Radiological Health, Malvina Eydelman, said "Early detection of retinopathy is an important part of managing care for the millions of people with diabetes, yet many patients with diabetes are not adequately screened for diabetic retinopathy since about 50 percent of them do not see their eye doctor on a yearly basis. Today's decision permits the marketing of a novel artificial intelligence technology that can be used in a primary care doctor's office. The FDA will continue to facilitate the availability of safe and effective digital health devices that may improve patient access to needed health care," (FDA 2018). The device is called IDx-DR and analyzes images of the eye taken with a retinal camera called the Topcon NW400. It therefore provides a screening decision without the need for a clinician to also interpret the image. The IDx-DR is the first of probably many other AI-powered tools to be approved by the FDA.

Many researchers have pointed to the smartphone as a great instrument to empower patients to manage their own health on a daily basis (Topol 2015; Insel 2017). In his book *The Patient Will See You Now*, Eric Topol even compared the smartphone invention to the introduction of mechanical movable type printing by Johannes Gutenberg in 1440. Gutenberg's press started the Printing Revolution and is regarded as a milestone of the second millennium. Before Gutenberg's invention only the highly affluent, nobility, and priests had access to manuscripts and could read. Smartphones may have the same impact since they can help provide patients with insights about their own health. There is much more computing power in a smartphone than in the building-sized computers from Turing's time. This paradigm shift can potentially lead the world to an era where knowledge is not just in the minds of trained experts, but rather in the hands of any ordinary person holding a smartphone or a similar general purpose device. As regards people's access to technology, the trends look positive. The number of smartphones in the world continues to grow, and is estimated to reach over six billion devices in circulation by the year 2020 (Kharpal 2017). Other devices are sure to play an important role, such as the smartwatch, sales of which, according to CCS Insight, should rise by 20% every year for the next 5 years (Lamkin 2018), thus becoming a possible key player in health tech initiatives. People who the health system cannot reach would most certainly benefit from a cheap, secure and fast approach to obtaining clinical insights. This puts patients first and democratizes health.

Smartphone devices will also enable information to be gathered and processed in real time providing us with digital phenotypes, which could potentially help us understand illnesses, including mental disorders, and to proactively treat patients (Insel 2017). Variations in symptoms or cognition are common between medical appointments in patients with mental disorders. However, when a patient or a caregiver is asked about symptoms during a clinical appointment, he or she tends to rely on the current symptoms and extrapolate this perspective to the whole period between the two appointments (Insel 2017). It is impossible for a professional to constantly assess a patient's condition in order to obtain better measures because of the costs involved, both in logistic and financial terms. Computers, however, have no such problem, in fact there is potential for the development of continuous real-time monitoring, while the clinician will have access to this information in graph format on his or her computer. Moreover, this is a time where everything is connected. We are increasingly purchasing products that are constantly listening to us and logging our every move. The Internet of Things has made it possible for us to connect devices that would otherwise be offline. From microwave to smoke detectors, every device in our house is, or could potentially be, gathering and logging our actions (Klous and Wielaard 2016). Through ubiquitous and pervasive computing, we are

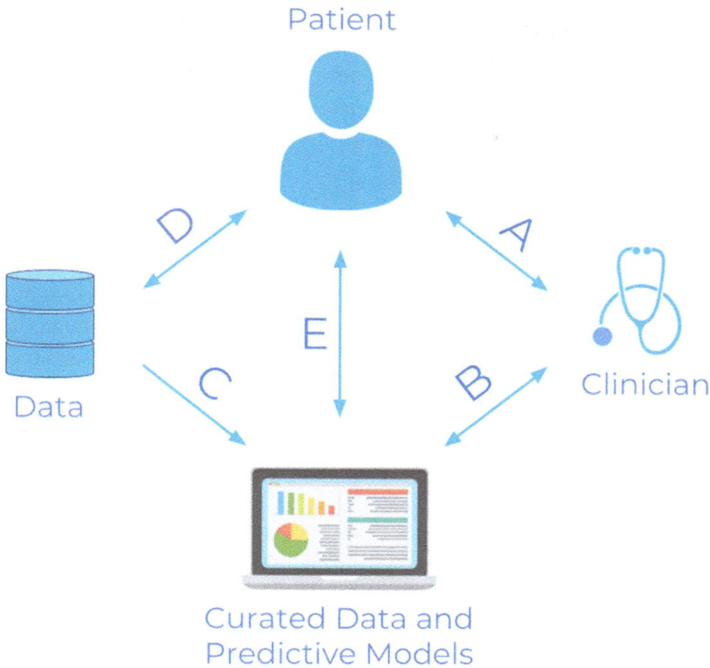

Fig. 1.3 The impact of big data coupled with advanced machine learning techniques may change the traditional doctor–patient relationship. (A) Traditional clinician–patient relationship: patients provide clinicians with the information that they need to diagnose and treat based on the judgment of the latter. (B) Clinical calculators: software-based clinical decision support systems built from machine-learning-based studies further improve the clinicians confidence in diagnosis and treatment. (C) Towards precise health care, curators may have access to data from the patient collected by multiple sensors and exams. The curators than proceed in creating a more friendly view of the data alongside predictive models that can assess diagnosis and prognosis of multiple conditions. Curators, in essence, are scientists and engineers with predictive modelling, health sciences, big data and analytic skills. (D) The patient owns all data, providing the control on sharing and how to proceed on its usage. (E) Patient self-assessment: Curated data and predictive models allow patients to receive clinical insights directly related to his/her diagnosis or prognosis and seek clinical evaluation if necessary. This shifts the passive role of the most interested in treatment, the patient, to an active role

also able to collect data without the patient realizing it; a good example is wearable technology, such as smartwatches, that can monitor a heart rate throughout the whole day. Putting aside for a moment the obvious security issues, these gadgets have great potential to assist clinical practice (Duffy et al. 2017). The information gathered between episodes could help us to understand better an individual patient's trends on multiple measures and personal idiosyncrasies. From the amount of time a patient spends on his or her smartphone to how s/he interacts with his or her personal assistant and social media, all could become digital biomarkers, which can be used by a clinician to assess a patient's behavior through predictive modelling. This kind of measurement paves the way for patients' empowerment. This would not remove the clinician from a patient's treatment, but rather would enable the patient to follow their health more closely and leave more complex decision making to the clinician. We believe that the traditional clinician–patient relationship will change with the introduction of big data and machine learning models. Figure 1.3 depicts how we see this development.

All these paradigm changes, ranging from individualized treatment to the collection and usage of data for patient self-assessment and clinical assistance, do not mean much if they are not put into practice. For that reason, we must change the way we observe predictive models and their impact to a more pragmatic point of view. In the next chapters, we will see how, from a clinical perspective, big data and machine learning will affect clinicians, addressing specifically mental health.

References

Bishop CM (2006) Pattern recognition and machine learning. Springer, Berlin

Cao B, Cho RY, Chen D et al (2018) Treatment response prediction and individualized identification of first-episode drug-naïve schizophrenia using brain functional connectivity. Mol Psychiatry. https://doi.org/10.1038/s41380-018-0106-5

Caspi A, McClay J, Moffitt TE et al (2002) Role of genotype in the cycle of violence in maltreated children. Science 297:851–854. https://doi.org/10.1126/science.1072290

Chekroud AM, Zotti RJ, Shehzad Z et al (2016) Cross-trial prediction of treatment outcome in depression: a machine learning approach. Lancet Psychiatry 3:243–250. https://doi.org/10.1016/S2215-0366(15)00471-X

Duffy A, Goodday S, Passos IC, Kapczinski F (2017) Changing the bipolar illness trajectory. Lancet Psychiatry 4:11–13. https://doi.org/10.1016/S2215-0366(16)30352-2

Evidence-Based Medicine Working Group (1992) Evidence-based medicine. A new approach to teaching the practice of medicine. JAMA 268:2420–2425

FDA (2018) Press Announcements - FDA permits marketing of artificial intelligence-based device to detect certain diabetes-related eye problems.https://www.fda.gov/newsevents/newsroom/pressannouncements/ucm604357.htm. Accessed 23 Aug 2018

Greenhalgh T, Howick J, Maskrey N (2014) Evidence based medicine: a movement in crisis. BMJ 348:g3725–g3725. https://doi.org/10.1136/bmj.g3725

Insel TR (2017) Digital phenotyping: technology for a new science of behavior. JAMA 318:1215–1216. https://doi.org/10.1001/jama.2017.11295

Kessler RC, Rose S, Koenen KC et al (2014) How well can post-traumatic stress disorder be predicted from pre-trauma risk factors? An exploratory study in the WHO world mental health surveys. World Psychiatry 13:265–274. https://doi.org/10.1002/wps.20150

Kharpal A (2017) Smartphone market worth $355 billion, with 6 billion devices in circulation by 2020: report. In: CNBC. https://www.cnbc.com/2017/01/17/6-billion-smartphones-will-be-in-circulation-in-2020-ihs-report.html . Accessed 28 Aug 2018

Klous S, Wielaard N (2016) We are big data: the future of the information society. Atlantis Press, Amsterdam

Lamkin P (2018) Smartwatch popularity booms with fitness trackers on the slide. In: Forbes. https://www.forbes.com/sites/paullamkin/2018/02/22/smartwatch-popularity-booms-with-fitness-trackers-on-the-slide/#20c9bb477d96. Accessed 28 Aug 2018

Leucht S, Cipriani A, Spineli L et al (2013) Comparative efficacy and tolerability of 15 antipsychotic drugs in schizophrenia: a multiple-treatments meta-analysis. Lancet 382:951–962. https://doi.org/10.1016/S0140-6736(13)60733-3

Librenza-Garcia D, Kotzian BJ, Yang J et al (2017) The impact of machine learning techniques in the study of bipolar disorder: a systematic review. Neurosci Biobehav Rev 80:538–554. https://doi.org/10.1016/j.neubiorev.2017.07.004

Lippi D, Gotuzzo E (2014) The greatest steps towards the discovery of Vibrio cholerae. Clin Microbiol Infect 20:191–195. https://doi.org/10.1111/1469-0691.12390

Mitchell TM (Tom M (1997) Machine learning. McGraw-Hill, New York

Mwangi B, Wu M-J, Cao B et al (2016) Individualized prediction and clinical staging of bipolar disorders using neuroanatomical biomarkers. Biol Psychiatry Cogn Neurosci Neuroimaging 1:186–194. https://doi.org/10.1016/j.bpsc.2016.01.001

Obermeyer Z, Emanuel EJ (2016) Predicting the future — big data, machine learning, and clinical medicine. N Engl J Med 375:1216–1219. https://doi.org/10.1056/NEJMp1606181

Passos IC, Mwangi B, Kapczinski F (2016) Big data analytics and machine learning: 2015 and beyond. Lancet Psychiatry 3:13–15. https://doi.org/10.1016/S2215-0366(15)00549-0

Pinto JV, Passos IC, Gomes F et al (2017) Peripheral biomarker signatures of bipolar disorder and schizophrenia: a machine learning approach. Schizophr Res 188:182–184. https://doi.org/10.1016/j.schres.2017.01.018

Robins L (1966) Deviant children grown up: a sociological and psychiatric study of sociopathic personality. Williams & Wilkins, Oxford

Sartori JM, Reckziegel R, Passos IC et al (2018) Volumetric brain magnetic resonance imaging predicts functioning in bipolar disorder: a machine learning approach. J Psychiatr Res 103:237–243. https://doi.org/10.1016/j.jpsychires.2018.05.023

Silver D, Schrittwieser J, Simonyan K et al (2017) Mastering the game of go without human knowledge. Nature 550:354–359. https://doi.org/10.1038/nature24270

Snow J (1854) The cholera near Golden Square and at Deptford. Med Times Gaz 9:321–322

Susser ES (2006) Psychiatric epidemiology: searching for the causes of mental disorders. Oxford University Press, Oxford

Susser M, Susser E (1996) Choosing a future for epidemiology: I. Eras and paradigms. Am J Public Health 86:668–673

Sutton RS, Barto AG (1998) Reinforcement learning: an introduction. MIT Press, Cambridge

TIME (2011) The 50 best inventions - TIME. http://content.time.com/time/subscriber/article/0,33009,2099708-11,00.html. Accessed 28 Aug 2018

Ting DSW, Cheung CY-L, Lim G et al (2017) Development and validation of a deep learning system for diabetic retinopathy and related eye diseases using retinal images from multiethnic populations with diabetes. JAMA 318:2211. https://doi.org/10.1001/jama.2017.18152

Topol EJ (2015) The patient will see you now: the future of medicine is in your hands. Basic Books, New York

Turing AM (1937) On computable numbers, with an application to the entscheidungsproblem. Proc Lond Math Soc s2–42(1):230–265

Turing AM (1950) Computing machinery and intelligence. Mind 49:433–460

Wu M-J, Mwangi B, Bauer IE et al (2017) Identification and individualized prediction of clinical phenotypes in bipolar disorders using neurocognitive data, neuroimaging scans and machine learning. NeuroImage 145:254–264. https://doi.org/10.1016/j.neuroimage.2016.02.016

Wu M-J, Passos IC, Bauer IE et al (2016) Individualized identification of euthymic bipolar disorder using the Cambridge neuropsychological test automated battery (CANTAB) and machine learning. J Affect Disord 192:219–225. https://doi.org/10.1016/j.jad.2015.12.053

2 Major Challenges and Limitations of Big Data Analytics

Bo Cao and Jim Reilly

Mental disorders have been considered as the top burden among global health problems, contributing about 32.4% years lived with disability (YLDs) and a cost of 2.5 trillion US dollars including both the direct and indirect costs (Vigo et al. 2016; Whiteford et al. 2013; Trautmann et al. 2016). The economic cost from mental disorders is expected to double by 2030. Because mental disorders usually appear early in the life, they may become a life-time burden for the patients and the caregivers. With the increasing number of patients in mental disorders and a growing aging population, the life burden and economic cost of mental disorders will be more than those of cardiovascular disease, common infections and cancer. However, unlike other physical diseases, we still highly rely on symptoms and do not have objective markers to make diagnosis of mental disorders. Once patients are diagnosed with mental disorders, we respond with a trial-and-error procedure to treat them. We seem to lack a good way to know the best treatment for a patient in advance and to provide optimal personalized treatment. These two major issues are pressing grand challenges to psychiatrists and researchers in the field of mental disorders.

The emerging field of "big data" in psychiatry opens a promising path to precise diagnosis and treatment of mental disorders. Over years of debating and hard work, researchers have come to an agreement that mental disorders are complicated and one disorder is probably not caused by a single change in the genes or neurons. However, by using high-dimensional data, such as genome-wide transcription and

B. Cao (✉)
Department of Psychiatry, Faculty of Medicine & Dentistry, University of Alberta, Edmonton, AB, Canada
e-mail: cloudbocao@gmail.com

J. Reilly
Department of Electrical and Computer Engineering, McMaster University, Hamilton, ON, Canada

I. C. Passos et al., *Personalized Psychiatry*,
https://doi.org/10.1007/978-3-030-03553-2_2

brain images, and integrating information from different modalities, we may be able to development methods of precise diagnosis and treatment prediction of mental disorders. Because the dimension of the data available is so high, a large number of observations are required correspondingly to develop and validate any model or method based on the data, which lead to a big volume of data with high dimensions and high instances. With the help of big data, it becomes possible to implement technics like data mining and machine learning to establish data-driven diagnoses and treatment strategies of mental disorders. Along with the opportunities brought by the big data in psychiatry are some unprecedented challenges.

In this chapter, we will name some challenges we are facing in the field of big data analytics in psychiatry. We hope to address and overcome these challenges with the joint force of researchers in related fields and alleviate the burden of mental disorders.

2.1 Challenges in Data Standardization

The data and knowledge shared should be scalable, expandable, transferrable and sustainable. This means that by increasing the volume of the data, we should achieve better performance of methods developed on the data and higher confidence of the outcomes, and we should be able the transfer the methods developed on one population to other populations and on the current generation to the future generations. One of the major challenges of big data analytics in psychiatry is that data collected globally is not always combinable due to the lack of standardization across regional centers and hospitals. Standardization can be considered as common features or measurements shared between datasets in the raw format in a strict sense. The measurements, or what data to collect, are usually determined upon an agreement across clinicians and researchers from different regions and disciplines. Standardization can also be considered as major shared information between datasets in a general sense. Even though the datasets may look different, the same features could be extracted after preprocessing. Lack of standardization is usually due to a disagreement among data collection parties, and makes it difficult to generalize the analysis based on one dataset to other datasets, or transfer the knowledge learned by the machine from one to another.

The first level of lack of standardization is from the diagnosis criteria. Although many researchers aim to move away from symptom-based diagnosis and achieve an objective diagnosis system based on biological markers, we still need to reply on the current diagnosis system to establish research samples. However, discrepancies in major diagnosis criteria across the world still exist. For example, bipolar disorder in children and adolescents is still diagnosed differently in Europe and U.S., resulting a much lower prevalence of bipolar disorder in Europe than U.S. (Soutullo and Chang 2005), and it is a debating topic whether bipolar disorder progresses or has severity stages (Berk et al. 2007; Passos et al. 2016; Cao et al. 2016; Kapczinski et al. 2016). Discrepancies of this kind will make it difficult to integrate data from different regions, as the data from patients with a certain label in one region may actually represent different populations in another region. It may also make it difficult the apply models developed with data from one region to those from another region, when these regions have different diagnosis criteria.

The changes of major diagnosis criteria over the years may also expose challenges in the consistency of the methods developed with data based on these criteria. For example, the data collected from patients with autism spectrum disorder (ASD) based on the fifth edition of Diagnostic and Statistical Manual of Mental Disorders (DSM; DSM-5) may include patients that were labeled as another disorder according to the fourth edition of DSM (DSM-IV). Patients that were considered to have obsessive-compulsive disorder (OCD) or posttraumatic stress disorder (PTSD) according to DSM-5 might share the same biological signatures of patients with anxiety disorders diagnosed according to DSM-IV (American Psychiatric Association 2013a, b). These changes of criteria are sometimes due to disagreement among the clinicians and researchers, but with good intention to provide better mental health services and to reflect recent progress in the research in mental disorders. The changes of criteria will be always a challenge for big data analytics in psychiatry, as it will be hard to keep tracks of findings based on different versions of the criteria. However, as more data are generated, shared and utilized, we believe that the criteria based on the biological markers will eventually emerge and converge with the criteria based on symptoms.

The second level of lack of standardization is from the different variables or modalities collected from regional data. Researchers have already realized the value of multi-modality data in psychiatry, which usually provide a more thorough understanding of mental disorder mechanisms and a better performance of computational models in making classifications and predictions of diagnosis and treatment responses compare to data of single modality. However, it is not always possible to collect all the crucial modalities. For example, magnetic resonance imaging (MRI) can provide non-invasive measurement of brain structure and functions in-vivo, and is a powerful tool for psychiatric research especially when combined with genetic measurements (Stein et al. 2011). However, a MRI scanner is luxury equipment for many hospitals in the developing countries, and many research projects may have to drop the MRI component due to the shortage of financial support even when the patient resource is sufficient. Some scanning procedures may require dedicated expertise, such as MR spectroscopy, advanced diffusion tensor imaging and scanning very young children or patients under states involving excessive head movements (Cao et al. 2017a), which may also become challenges for hospitals and research centers without corresponding supports.

Different variables, assessments and outcome indicators may also be used in electronic health records (EHR) and health information (HI) across regions and nations. It is quite common that even with the same diagnosis criteria, clinicians and health service providers from different regions or countries may have different interpretations of the criteria and different ways to record cases. They may also add their own insight or adapt a general procedure to meet the need of local populations. All these variations of recording the patient information may lead to various measurements that are unique to certain data collection, which will cause difficulty when a method developed on one dataset is being transferred or applied to another dataset. The EHR and HI are emerging technology in mental health, and each country is still trying to implement them efficiently according to its own medical, privacy, political and financial environments. However, it is important for researchers and policy makers to realize the necessity to facilitate a communicable and compatible health record system for the future global effort in mental health research.

The third level of lack of standardization is from varies of protocols in data collection. Although some datasets shared the same variables, they may show quite significant difference in the same variables due to different protocols of data collections, storage and preprocessing. For example, in a large multi-center neuroimaging dataset, the study site is one of the most significant contributors to the variance even in some of the basic measurements like cortical and subcortical region volumes (Panta et al. 2016). The effect of the study sites may be attributed to several sources, such as different brands of scanners, scanning sequences and parameters, preprocessing pipelines and even different instructions for the patients. Since it is not possible to use the same scanner and technicians to perform all the data collection, one strategy could be using common phantoms across study sites and follow the protocol in a well-established large-sample study, such as the human connectome project (http://www.humanconnectomeproject.org). Another strategy is to include a well-represented sample of healthy subjects that serves as the reference when the measurements of current dataset are compared to other public datasets (Cao et al. 2017b). The difference in the measurements between the healthy subjects in different datasets could be used to calibrate the corresponding measurements for all the subjects including patients and healthy subjects, so that different patient populations from different datasets can be compared directly (Fig. 2.1).

Another challenge in data standardization is the fast evolving technics in biology, imaging and computational analysis. We are in such a fast pace in the development of new technologies in biology and the ways that we can measure the genes, neurons, brain anatomy, networks and functions are evolving every day. New standard measurements that were not possible or affordable are being introduced more frequently than ever. Thus, it is a great challenge for us to think ahead when new data collection is planned. It is also important to keep updating and correcting knowledge derived from data collected previously. A result no matter how intuitive at the time of publication could be found less accurate when a new method is developed. For example, the segmentation of hippocampal subfields were found to be less accurate in an older version of method compared to the new version (Andreasen et al. 2011; Cao et al. 2017c, 2018), and findings using the previous version of method need to be updated and interpreted with caution (Van Leemput et al. 2009; Haukvik et al. 2015). For another example, researchers have generally believed that there is no lymphatic system in our brain, until very recently some study confirmed that our brain actually has a lymphatic system to circulate immune cells and wastes using advanced MRI imaging technics (Absinta et al. 2017). This will not only change the textbooks about the lymphatic system, but will also bring

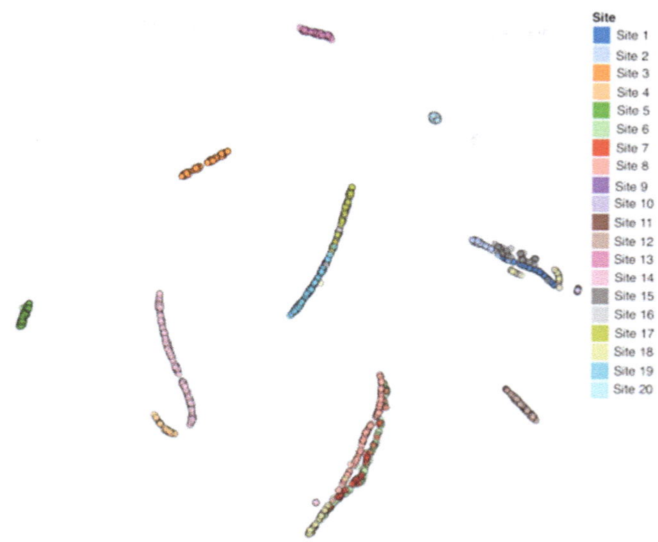

Fig. 2.1 Effect from study sites in a large sample multi-center neuroimaging study. Adapted from Panta et al. (2016)

new possible measurements about brain immunometabolism in mental disorders involving altered immune activities like neural or glial inflammation.

Although it is convenient to have the exact same measurements in datasets collected across regions for the purpose of implementing many machine learning algorithms and analyses, the advance of computational algorithms may provide more tolerance of less standardized data. Traditional methods, such as support vector machines (SVM) and regularized linear regressions have made substantial progress in big data analytics in psychiatry. However, they may require relatively strict standardization across the datasets when a model using them needs to be generalized and transferred from one dataset to another dataset. New progress in deep learning networks may relieve some of the restrictions in the variables collected in different datasets because methods like deep learning may involve an integrated feature learning process that does not need the raw data to be in the exact form from different datasets (Rajkomar et al. 2018). New computational algorithms may help to automatically "standardize" features from different variables in different datasets, and make it easy to transfer models across datasets.

The challenges due to lack of standardization could be partly overcome with good strategic planning and collaboration between developed and developing regions. The data and methods shared in the research community have made substantial contribution to the progress of mental disorder research and brain research in general. A transparent ecology to share the lessons learned during the data collection and sharing, and an open environment to facilitate the agreement on the variables and protocols in patient evaluation and data collection will advance the progress in big data analytics in psychiatry.

2.2 Challenges in Machine Learning in Psychiatry

2.2.1 Overview of Machine Learning in Psychiatry

The machine learning (ML) paradigm is the new frontier in brain health research. The brain is far too complicated an organism to enable modeling by classical means, a process which would typically involve the use of mathematical and physical constructs or laws to predict brain *behaviour* in some way. However, our understanding of the brain is currently at such an underdeveloped state that we as humans know of no encompassing set of physical and mathematical laws that can adequately describe brain behaviour over a wide range of circumstances. In fact, the concept of humans trying to understand their own brains is a conundrum, well expressed by Emerson Pugh in the early 1930s: *"If the human brain were so simple that we could understand it, we would be so simple that we couldn't."*

Fortunately however, the machine learning paradigm allows us to circumvent this difficulty, at least in part. Machine learning can be used to construct a rudimentary model that can predict behaviour of a complex system in a limited sense. The machine learning model compares measurements describing a system under test with previous measurements of similar systems whose behaviour has been observed and is therefore known. Because the machine learning method can then predict behavior of the complex system, it in essence constructs a rudimentary model of the system itself.

We now give a simple example of how a machine learning model can be developed that could train a "Man from Mars" to distinguish whether a particular human specimen is male or female. In this problem, there are two *classes*; male and female. We must first have available a set of N humans and their corresponding male/female class labels. Since the Man from Mars has very little prior knowledge about distinguishing male humans from female humans, he assembles a large group of measurements (*features*) from each human sample. This list of features (referred to as the *candidate features*) are only his guesses of which measurements might be discriminative between the classes. Let us say the candidate features he chooses in this case are hair length, number of teeth, skin colour, voice pitch, and weight. These candidate features are fed into a *feature selection* algorithm (to be described later) that identifies only those features which are discriminative between the classes. We observe that skin colour, number of teeth, and to some extent weight, have little bearing in determining gender. So the feature selection algorithm selects hair length and voice pitch from the list of candidate features. (We prefer only two features so we can plot in 2 dimensions). We can interpret these features as axes in a Cartesian coordinate space (called the *feature space*), and then plot the corresponding hair length and voice pitch values for each of our N human samples as a point in this feature space, as shown in Fig. 2.2. We see that the points representing the male

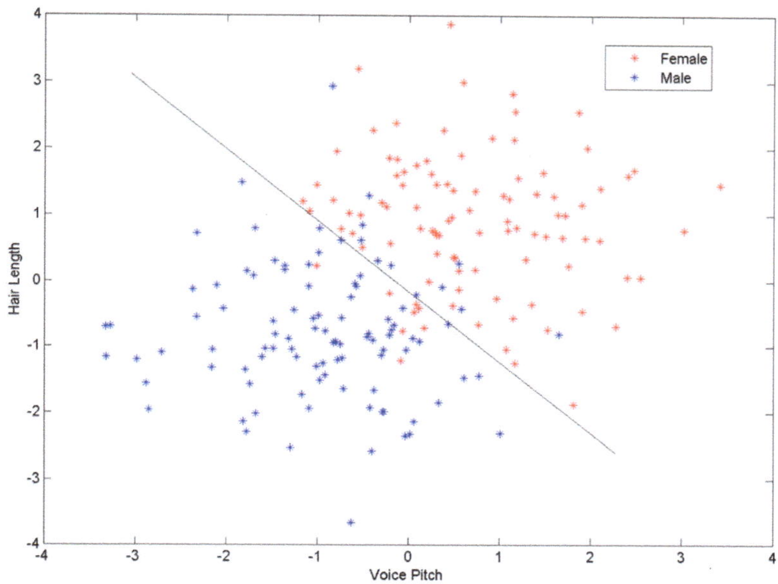

Fig. 2.2 Feature space for the "Man from Mars" example

and female samples tend to cluster into two distinct regions in the sample space—females in the upper right, and males in the lower left.

We then design a *classifier*, which in this simple case is a straight line that separates the two classes as cleanly as possible. Now that our Man from Mars has his rudimentary model constructed, he can determine the gender of a previously unseen human by measuring their hair length and voice pitch and plot the corresponding point in the feature space. The gender is determined by which side of the line the point falls on.

Let the number of selected features be M. The M features collected from each of the available N humans may be assembled into N vectors $\boldsymbol{x}_n, n = 1, \ldots, N$, each of which is of dimension $(M \times 1)$. Let us denote the corresponding (binary) class label for each human (sample) as y_n. Then the set $(\boldsymbol{x}_n, y_n), n = 1, \ldots, N$ is called the *training set*.

Our Man may wish to determine the accuracy of his rudimentary machine learning model. He may accomplish this using a *validation procedure*, which is an essential part of the machine learning process.

In Fig. 2.2 we see that some samples from each class fall on the wrong side of the boundary. This is because in this case there are some men with long hair and high voices and women with short hair and low voices. Misclassification is unavoidable in most machine learning problems; however we wish to minimize this effect by choosing the best possible combination of features and the best possible classification rule.

Thus we see there are three major components of a machine learning modelling process; these are feature selection, classification and validation. We discuss each of these components more thoroughly in the sequel, with a view to how each of the respective algorithms behave in applications related to psychiatry and neuroscience.

2.2.2 Feature Selection, Classification, and Validation Algorithms

2.2.2.1 The Feature Selection Process

In typical applications in psychiatry and neuroscience, and in many medical applications in general, the number of candidate features tends to be large but the number of available training samples is few. This scenario is difficult for the machine learning paradigm, since according to Bellman's "curse of dimensionality"(Bellman and Dreyfus 1962), the number of training samples required to maintain classification performance at a specified level grows exponentially with the number of features used by the classifier. So to maintain satisfactory levels of classification accuracy, especially in the presence of few training samples, we require the number of features adopted by the machine learning model to be as small as possible. As we have seen previously, this is accomplished using a feature selection process.

Feature selection methods, in the general sense, identify features which have a high level of statistical dependency with the class label. This means the values of selected features change significantly with class. Another interpretation of feature selection is in the *data compression*, or *dimensionality reduction* context. That is, a feature selection process identifies features which preserve the underlying characteristics of the data with as high fidelity as possible using as few features as possible.

One of the issues worthy of consideration in feature selection is that it is necessary to examine the relevance of *groups* of features rather than just features individually. An example is shown in Fig. 2.3 where it is seen that each feature individually is not discriminative; however, when considered jointly the two classes separate cleanly. Thus, an ideal feature selection algorithm must examine all possible combinations of all available N candidate features for relevance. This is a problem with combinatorial complexity and so is computationally intractable. We must therefore resort to a suboptimal approach for selecting features if we are to circumvent these computational difficulties. In practice, all practical feature selection approaches are suboptimal in some sense.

Feature selection is an intensively studied topic and accordingly there are a very large number of feature selection algorithms available in the literature. An extensive list of modern feature selection methods is provided in Armanfard et al. (2017). A feature selection method that has proven to be very effective in applications related to brain research is the minimum redundancy maximum relevance (mRMR) method (Peng et al. 2005). The mRMR method uses *mutual information* as a measure of statistical dependency. It is an iterative greedy approach where in each iteration a single feature is chosen which has the maximum mutual information with the class labels (relevance) but minimum mutual information (redundancy) with the set of

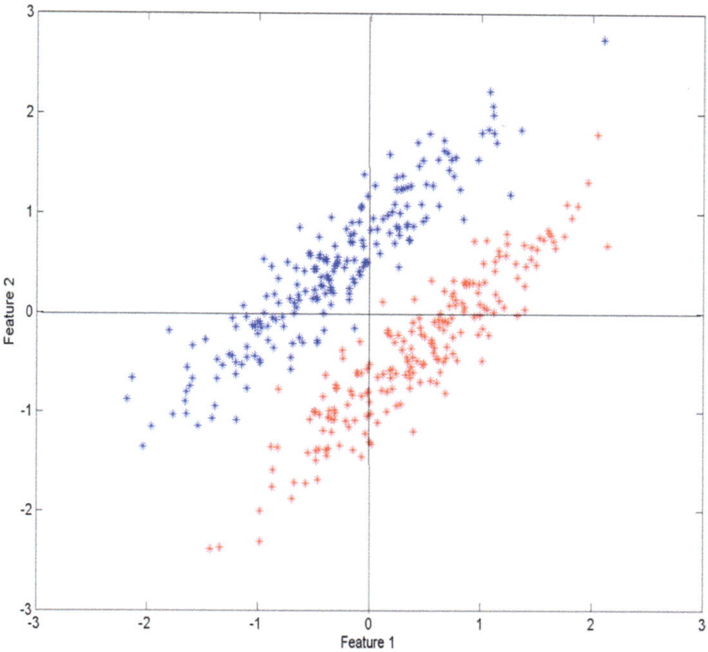

Fig. 2.3 A feature space in 2 dimensions, where neither feature is discriminative on its own, yet jointly they are highly discriminative

features chosen in previous iterations. C code for the mRMR method is available on line at http://home.penglab.com/p_publication.html.

Often in feature selection problems, the scale of the candidate features can vary over many orders of magnitude. This extensive range of values can pose difficulties for the feature selection and classification algorithms. This issue may be conveniently resolved by normalizing the values of each feature using e.g. their z-score. That is, all values x_{mn} of the mth feature are replaced with the value $x'_{mn} = \frac{x_{mn} - u_m}{\sigma_m}, n = 1, \ldots, N$, where μ_m and σ_m are the mean and standard deviation respectively of the mth feature evaluated over the N available samples from the training set.

2.2.2.2 The Classification Process

The features are selected so that the samples from each class in the training set separate (i.e. cluster) as well as possible into two (in the binary case) distinct regions in the feature space, each region corresponding to a class. In a typical machine learning scenario, the two classes seldom separate cleanly; there is usually some overlap between the clusters representing each of the classes. The classifier may be described as a mathematical rule that maps a prescribed (i.e. test) point in the feature space into a class, in some optimal fashion that minimizes the occurrence of a classification error. That is, the classifier determines the most likely cluster that a test point belongs to. Note that points which fall into an overlap region between clusters may not classify correctly.

There are many types of classifier. The support vector machine (SVM) (Haykin 2009; Hastie et al. 2009) is a well-established classification method that has been shown to behave well in psychiatric applications, with a built in SVM function available in later versions of Matlab and Tensor Flow. The basic version of the SVM classifier formulates a hyperplane that separates the two classes so that the *margin* is maximized. The margin is the distance from the closest points in each class to the hyperplane. These closest points are referred to as *support vectors*; hence the name of the classifier.

Classification is a very mature topic and consequently there are many types of classification methods, in addition to the SVM, that are available in the literature. Examples include *K* Nearest Neighbor (KNN), the Linear Discriminant Analyzer (LDA), the naïve Bayes classifier, decision trees, etc. These are all described in Hastie et al. (2009). There is also the well-known multi-layer perceptron as described in Rumelhart (1986) and Haykin (2009).

Decision trees are specifically useful in the present context since they form the basis of more sophisticated classifiers which we discuss later in this section. There are several tree-based training methods that are discussed in Hastie et al. (2009) and Bishop (2006). A characteristic of the decision tree is that it produces unbiased outputs with high variance; hence, they are not useful as is for classification.

Classifiers, as well as many feature selection algorithms, usually have at least one associated parameter whose value must be tuned to produce optimal classification performance in a given scenario. For example, the SVM classifier incorporates a user-defined parameter that controls the tradeoff between increasing the margin size and ensuring that the training sample feature vectors $\mathbf{x}_\mathrm{n}$ lie on the correct side of the margin. Another example is the parameter *K* (number of nearest neighbours) in the KNN classifier. Details on how to select a suitable value for these parameters are described in Sect. 13.2.2.3.

Classification in the Nonlinearly Separable Case: In Figs. 2.2 and 2.3, we have shown simple cases where the class clusters separate linearly. While this is the easiest case to deal with from the theoretical perspective, in practice the boundaries between the classes are seldom linear, as shown in the example on the left in Fig. 2.4. In this case, it can be seen that if a linear boundary is used to separate the feature space on the left, significant classification error will result.

Fortunately, under certain conditions, various forms of classifier like the SVM can be easily adopted to the nonlinear boundary case using the so-called *kernel trick* e.g., Bishop (2006). The kernel trick is applicable if the only numerical operations performed by the classifier are inner products. The kernel trick in effect maps the original data in the original Cartesian space through a nonlinear transformation Φ into a higher-dimensional space where ideally, the data separate linearly, as shown on the right in Fig. 2.4. The interesting feature of the kernel trick however is that the nonlinear transformation is not performed explicitly. Instead, it may be induced simply by replacing each inner product operation of the form $\boldsymbol{x}^T\boldsymbol{z}$ involved in the

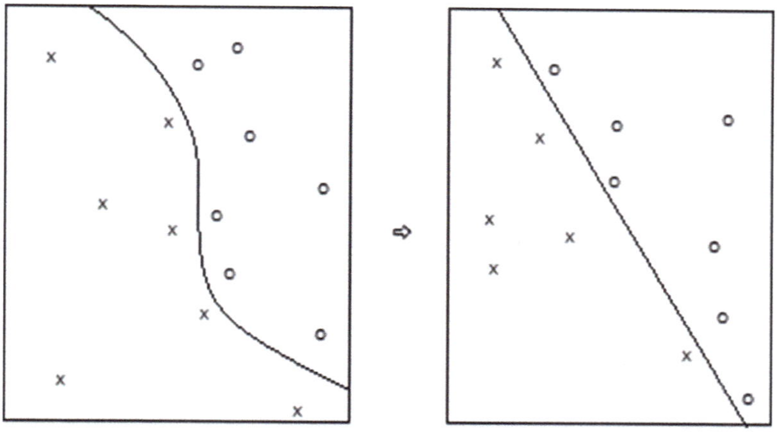

Fig. 2.4 Transformation of a nonlinear feature space (left) in to a linear separable space (right)

implementation of the classifier algorithm with a kernel function $k(\boldsymbol{x}, z)$,where $\boldsymbol{x}$ and z are feature vectors in the present case.

Kernel functions can be interpreted as similarity measures; the larger the value of the function, the more similar are the vector arguments **x** and **z**. They must obey the property that its associated Gram matrix be positive definite. Examples of valid kernel functions are the Gaussian kernel $k(\boldsymbol{x}, z) = \exp\left(-\gamma||\boldsymbol{x} - z||_2^2\right)$,where γ is a real-valued user-defined parameter, and the polynomial kernel $k(\boldsymbol{x}, z) = (\boldsymbol{x}^T z + c)^d$, where c and d are also real-valued user-defined parameters. The respective parameters are adjusted so that the boundary in the transformed space is as linear as possible. More details on all aspects of the kernelization process are available in Müller et al. (2001) and Bishop (2006).

Machine Learning Methods Specifically Recommended for Use in Brain Research The first such approach which has proven useful in brain studies is the mRMR feature selection scheme in conjunction with an SVM classifier (Khodayari-Rostamabad et al. 2010, 2013; Ravan et al. 2011, 2012; Colic et al. 2017). For example, in Khodayari-Rostamabad et al. (2013) this approach was used to predict response of patients with major depressive disorder to treatment with an SSRI.

Adaboost Another approach uses *boosting* (Bishop 2006) where the idea is to aggregate many "weak" classifiers (learners) into one that is very "strong". The *Adaboost* algorithm (Schapire 2003) is a well-known example of such a method. This method uses multiple instances of weak learners. For training, each weak classifier weighs each sample of the training set differently, with more weight being placed on the samples which the classifiers get wrong. The Adaboost algorithm combines the feature selection and classification roles and typically uses decision trees as the weak learner. It forms its final output decision on a majority vote amongst the weak learners. The Adaboost algorithm has the desirable property that, provided the individual weak learners give better than chance accuracy, then the probability of error of the aggregate classifier decays exponentially as the number of learners increases (Schapire 2003).

Random Forest An additional (related) concept is *bagging*, which is short form for "aggregate bootstrapping". A widely used classification algorithm in this respect is the *random forest* (RF) classifier (Hastie et al. 2009; Breiman and Spector 1992). Like Adaboost, the RF classifier uses a multiplicity of decision trees, and again the final output decision is based on a majority vote over the individual decision trees. Unlike Adaboost, the input to each decision tree for training is a resampled (with replacement) version of the complete training set, and the feature inputs at each node are also randomly chosen. The RF classifier has the advantage that, unlike the other forms of classifier we have discussed so far, it is insensitive to the overfitting phenomenon, to be discussed later. It too combines the feature selection and classification processes. The RF classifier has been successfully used e.g. in detecting onset of epileptic ictal periods (Colic et al. 2017).

The Localized Feature Selection Method (LFS) Conventional forms of feature selection methods are global; i.e., they assign a single set of features that attempts to characterize the entire sample (i.e. training sample) space. In contrast, the LFS method (Armanfard et al. 2016a, 2017) allows the choice of selected features to vary across the sample space, thus adapting to variations such as nonlinearities, discontinuities or nonstationarities that may appear across different regions of the sample space. Each training sample is treated as a representative point for its surrounding region and as such is assigned its own distinct set of features. These (local) feature sets are determined by solving a straightforward optimization procedure in the form of a linear program. The LFS method, unlike deep learning methods, is therefore very easy to train. The LFS method is well suited to the "data poor" case where the number of candidate features far exceeds the number of available training samples, and is also immune to the overfitting problem (to be discussed). The LFS method has proven to be successful in predicting emergence in coma patients (Armanfard et al. 2016b).

There are also deep learning methods (Le Roux and Bengio 2008) that are currently a very active area of research. In particular, autoencoders (Le 2015) have the desirable characteristic of being able to automatically generate features directly from the data. Deep learning methods have been very successful in many applications; however, generally they require large, noise-free training sets. In many applications in psychiatry and related fields training data is very hard to come by, and so deep learning methods have not proven very successful for the applications at hand. It is for this reason they are not considered further in this chapter.

2.2.2.3 Validation and Measurement of Performance

Validation is a very important component of the machine learning model. It is used in conjunction with the available training set to determine classification accuracy of a proposed machine learning implementation. It is also instrumental in tuning the parameters that are associated with the feature identification, classification or kernelization procedures.

Before we discuss validation per se, we consider two different forms of error associated with the machine learning model. These are *training error* and *generalization* error. Training error is the classification error using the training set itself. An example is shown in Fig. 2.2. In this case, because of the overlap between the classes in the training set, we see that a linear boundary (as determined e.g. by an SVM) cannot separate the two classes without error. Generalization error on the other hand arises if a new sample which is not contained in the training set is incorrectly classified. The validation process estimates the generalization error of the respective machine learning model based on the training error.

The usual form of validation is *cross-validation*, where the available training set is split into two parts—the larger which is referred to as a *training set*, and the other the *test set*. The machine learning model is built using only the data in the training set. The performance of the resulting model is then evaluated by feeding the test set samples into the classifier and comparing the classification results with the corresponding labels provided by the test set.

The most common method is k-fold cross validation. Here the entire training set is partitioned into k contiguous groups, with each group containing the integer closest to N/k samples. The procedure iterates k times, where in each iteration one group is held out for testing and the remaining groups are used for training. Each group is left out once. The fold error is the average error rate over the samples in the group, and the overall error rate is the average of the group error. Leave-one-out cross validation (LOOCV) is a form of k-fold cross validation, except there are $k = N$ folds (i.e. there is only one sample in each test group). LOOCV works well in the small N case, but often is computationally expensive because the entire modelling process must be repeated N times. The method can be susceptible to high variance in the generalization error estimate. A third form of validation is bootstrapping. It is similar to k-fold cross validation except that in each fold the training and test groups are chosen randomly with replacement.

As discussed in Hastie et al. (2009), the cross-validation estimate of the generalization error is subject to both bias and variance. Bias happens because the number of training samples available in each fold may be inadequate to train the underlying model accurately. This results in the cross-validation procedure over-estimating the generalization error. There is also a variance associated with the cross-validation estimate, since it is obtained by averaging over a finite number of samples. As k decreases, the variance increases but the bias decreases. Breiman and Spector (1992) and Kohavi (1995) suggest that a value of $k = 5$ or 10 gives a reasonable compromise between these two counter-acting effects.

A cross validation procedure can also be used to tune the parameters of the machine learning model. For example, if we are using a k-fold process for performance evaluation, the data in the training set in each fold is subjected to a second, inner cross-validation loop. In each fold of the inner loop, the data is again split into a "tuning" set and a test set. The inner loop is repeated several times using different values of the parameter, and the value giving the best performance is then selected for that fold of the outer loop.

A very important consideration in cross validation is that the training and test sets be kept completely separate. If a data sample is included in the training set and then afterwards is again used for testing, then performance is biased upwards, because the machine learning model has been specifically trained to avoid errors over *all* samples in the training data.

As an example of the machine learning process in psychiatry applications, we now briefly describe a study (Khodayari-Rostamabad et al. 2013) which used machine learning to predict response to SSRI treatment for major depressive disorder, based on analysis of the EEG. The training set consisted of EEG measurements from 22 patients who were diagnosed with MDD and whose response to the treatment was recorded after several months of treatment. The set of candidate features consisted of power spectral density measurements at many frequency values from all electrodes, and spectral coherence values from all pairs of electrodes over the same set of frequency values. The study used 20 electrodes and 50 frequency values, which resulted in over 10,000 candidate features. The mRMR feature selection algorithm was used to reduce this set down to 10 or fewer features which have the most relevance with the recorded response to the treatment. An SVM classifier was used and the estimated correct classification rate was approximately 85%. This study therefore provides a good indication that machine learning methods can adequately predict response using EEG analysis.

2.2.3 Further Considerations in the Development of a Machine Learning Model

2.2.3.1 The Over/Underfitting Problem

Consider the situation shown in Fig. 2.2 where a linear boundary does not cleanly separate the training samples into their respective classes. The temptation in this case may be to build a classifier that that can generate a more flexible boundary that works its way around the misfit points and so places the misplaced samples on the correct side of the boundary. This increased flexibility can be achieved by introducing additional parameters into the classifier model. In this case, the classifier can be trained so that the training error reduces to zero. Let us assume that the underlying true but unknown boundary corresponding to the physical process that generates the data is in fact linear. Then new data points placed where the flexible boundary has been diverted may not classify properly, and so the generalization error degrades in this case. This phenomenon is called *overfitting* and is a result of the machine learning model over-adapting to the training set (i.e. the boundary is allowed to become too "wiggly").

Another form of overfitting occurs when the dimension of the feature space becomes too large in proportion to the number of training samples. For example, in the linearly separable case, an n-dimensional hyperplane can always separate any arbitrary class configuration of $n + 1$ data points. So as the number of features increases, the classifier has more freedom to fit the training data, which implies the training error decreases, but at the cost of increased generalization error. It is fortunate that a properly executed cross-validation procedure will detect the presence of overfitting.

Underfitting occurs when the model is not flexible enough to fit the data. This could happen for example when the number of selected features is too small to adequately separate the training set. An example of the underfitting problem is as follows. Suppose we have a data set which separates cleanly with three features. In this case a classifier algorithm such as SVM would specify a boundary plane in the corresponding 3 dimensional space to separate the classes. Suppose now that we discarded one of the features used only two of the three features. Then all the data would be projected onto the remaining 2 dimensional plane and the two classes may overlap with each other, thus reducing performance.

If the number of features is too large, we have overfitting, and if too small, we have underfitting. So how to choose a good value? One valid method is to repetitively train a machine learning model for an increasing number of features (starting e.g. at 1) and test each model using a cross-validation procedure. We should see the error decrease initially as the number of features increases, because underfitting becomes less of an issue. But then as the number increases further, the error will bottom out to a plateau, and then begin to increase, due to overfitting. The best number of features to use may be taken as that corresponding to the minimum error.

2.2.3.2 Missing Data

In many applications, particularly in medicine, the feature vector associated with a specific data sample may not contain all the values or measurements of the specified selected features. When data is collected during studies, missing data may result from patient incompliance, patient drop-out, measurements being too inconvenient or expensive to acquire, etc. The problem is that many machine learning algorithms will not execute properly when some data from the feature vectors are missing. Thus some value for the missing features must be supplied in order for the algorithm to run properly on a computer. The problem is that an improperly substituted value for a missing value may adversely impact the accuracy of the machine learning model. So what value do we supply that will minimize this impact?"

There are many approaches available to address this question. One is simply to delete any incomplete samples. However, in doing so, we are throwing away useful data, and so this is an undesirable option. Other approaches therefore attempt to estimate suitable values for the missing features, based on the available remaining data. The process of filling in missing data is generally referred to as *imputation*. There are many forms of imputation, many of which are well discussed in García-Laencina et al. (2010). The basic idea behind imputation is that the statistical dependencies that may exist between the different feature values in a training sample are exploited to estimate the missing value. The difficulty with this approach is that in some cases, e.g., the mRMR method, the features are specifically selected so that the statistical dependencies between feature values is minimized. Thus in some cases imputation is an ineffective method.

In cases where there is significant correlation between feature values in a data sample, we can use ordinary regression to impute the missing data. Another approach is to use more sophisticated model-building statistical methods such as the EM algorithm. Yet another approach is to use a second-level machine learning approach to estimate the missing data in the primary problem. These methods are all discussed well in García-Laencina et al. (2010).

Perhaps the most sensible approach to handle the missing data case is to use feature selection and classification methods that can be adapted to tolerate missing data. Two such methods are the random forest (RF) and the localized feature selection (LFS) approach. When some features in the training set are missing, the training procedure for both algorithms is easily modified to accommodate this case. However, when testing data contains missing values, both models may have to be partially re-trained so that missing features in the test data are excluded. This can be expensive from the computational perspective, but the data imputation process involves a significant computational cost as well. At this point it is not known how the performance of the RF or LFS approaches to handling missing data compare to that of imputation methods. However, in the case where there is little statistical dependency between the selected feature values, the LFS and RF methods will almost surely perform better than methods using imputation.

2.2.3.3 Imbalanced Data

The data imbalance problem occurs when the training set consists of many more samples of one class than another. These are referred to as the majority vs. minority classes, respectively. For example, if a research study involves testing the human population at large for psychiatric illness, we are likely to find far more healthy subjects than ill patients. Thus the training set becomes imbalanced. Imbalanced data sets become a problem in the machine learning context, since the model is hindered in learning the distributive properties of the minority class. For example, in a case where the split between the majority vs. minority classes in the training set is 90% vs. 10%, the model need only output a majority class decision in all cases and overall, it would be correct 90% of the time. However, in this case the minority class would be misclassified 100% of the time. As a further example, studies (Woods et al. 1993) have been performed where machine learning was used to detect cancer from a mammography data set. The data set contained a 40:1 imbalance in favour of the noncancerous class. The results showed accuracy rates of close to 100% for the noncancerous case, and only approximately 10% for the cancerous class. Thus a large proportion of cancerous cases would be incorrectly classified as noncancerous. This case has more severe consequences than incorrectly diagnosing a noncancerous patient. This example illustrates that in the imbalanced data case, it is necessary to consider more refined performance metrics, such as receiver operating characteristic (ROC) curves and others that can weigh errors from the different classes in different degrees (He and Garcia 2009).

The negative consequences of the imbalanced data case become more severe when the class distributions in the feature space become more complex. This could happen e.g., if the distribution of one or both of the classes devolves into multiple clusters, or a single cluster of complex shape, instead of the ideal case where each class is represented by a single well-defined cluster. The situation is particularly severe in the high-dimensional case with few training data, since then there are not enough samples for the model to learn the characteristics of the minority class.

There are effective methods that have been developed to mitigate the imbalanced data problem. One such method that has shown a great deal of success in many applications is the synthetic minority oversampling technique (SMOTE) (Chawla et al. 2002). It balances the dataset by sampling (generating) synthetic minority class samples, and discarding some majority class samples, if necessary. The synthetic minority class samples are generated by selecting a specific minority class training sample at random. Artificial samples are generated by placing a new sample on a straight line between the minority sample under consideration and one of its K nearest neighbours of the same class. This sampling process can be repeated many times to generate as many synthetic minority class samples as desired. This method preserves the characteristics of the minority class data and has been demonstrated to work well in many situations. There are several variations on the basic method, as discussed in He and Garcia (2009). The SMOTE algorithm is included in the Tensorflow package.

The SMOTE method and its variants use sampling techniques to augment minority class samples. Another approach at handling the imbalanced data case are *cost-sensitive* methods, which effectively place more weight on minority class errors than on majority class errors during the training process. In many cases this can be achieved simply by trading off an increase in majority class error for an improvement in minority class performance. The Adaboost and LFS algorithms in particular are easily adapted to incorporate this tradeoff. In the Adaboost case, it is only necessary to modify the formulation of the distribution function over the training samples; with LFS, the tradeoff can be implemented simply by varying the parameter γ (Armanfard et al. 2016a, 2017). The literature on this topic is extensive; there is an abundant reference list in He and Garcia (2009).

2.3 Challenges from Data to Knowledge

Traditional ways of research in psychiatry tend to be reductionism and hypothesis driven, which is proved to be effective to investigate single-factor mechanism at the group-level. This approach is still the golden standard when it comes to establish the causality between a factor and the outcome, because we usually could only manipulate one or limited number of factors in experimental or clinical setups. When many factors, including genetic, physiological and behavioral factors, and their interactions need to be considered at the same time, it is usually not efficient, if not impossible, to use the reductionism approach to investigate one by one of the many possible factor combinations (Williams and Auwerx 2015). The new big data approach could take into account all the factors without many priori assumptions, which will lead to effective outcome prediction at the individual level and new hypotheses that have been ignored previously. This approach will provide translational applications in personalized psychiatry, as the knowledge or algorithms learned from existing data could be applied on new cases. It will also provide insights of important factors and their links in mental disorders, which can then be investigated using a hypothesis-driven approach. Thus, the traditional approach and the novel big data approach are complementary to each other in future research of mental disorders.

It is still crucial to transform the complex data with understandable representation in low dimensions in many cases, because we can visualize the data in 2D and 3D dimensions, static or changing over time. Visualization will help us to see high-dimensional data in an intuitive space. It will show data distributions for certain measurements and overlay measurements onto each other to show their interactions, which will help to understand the mechanisms underlying different measurements, identify the outliers and unusual cases, discover major variance contributors, select subsets of data for post-hoc analysis and so on. Although most of these tasks could also be done with proper mathematical tools directly applied at the high-dimensional data, it is challenging to make sense of the data when the dimension of the data is high and data involve multiple modalities. Moreover, visualization in low dimension is helpful for researchers to demonstrate certain concepts and convey the knowledge to the audience without professional data science training, such as some clinicians and patients. For example, a visualization method called t-distributed stochastic neighbor embedding (t-SNE) can help researchers see a large sample of high-dimensional multi-modal brain imaging data (Panta et al. 2016). We can easily see the reliable difference between images from 1.5 and 3 T scanners, and there seems to be no apparent difference in the scanning time. These observations may provide further confidence for us to combine existing images scanned at varied time of the day or to plan new scans without much concern of scanning time, while make us to be cautious about data that have been scanned or are going to be scanned with different magnetic field intensities. Big data visualization is still an emerging field and psychiatry will benefit from the development of it, yet it is also a challenging field with respect to the number of factors that need to be considered in mental health.

Big data in psychiatry armed with advanced machine learning and artificial intelligence technics will become one of the strongest tools in the research of mental disorders. However, as an interdisciplinary field, the collaboration between experts in psychiatry, neuroscience, psychology, computer science, mathematicians, and software engineers is not replaceable by the novel methods of big data analytics. The value of big data will not be appreciated by the public until it is converted to massive knowledge of mechanisms of mental disorders or translational tools that can guide the diagnosis and treatment of mental disorders. It is only when the interdisciplinary experts make joint forces together that the big data in psychiatry can reach its full potential to become beneficial knowledge and the corresponding challenges that we have discussed can be overcome (Fig. 2.5).

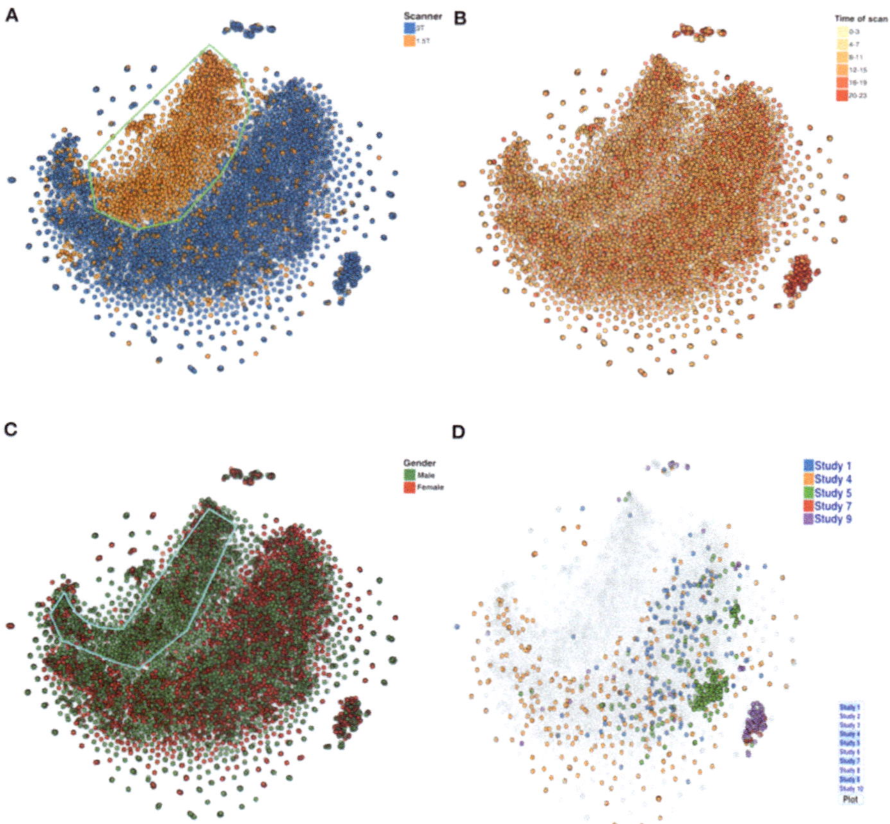

Fig. 2.5 t-SNE plots color coded by (**a**) scanner type (**b**) scan acquisition time (**c**) gender, and (**d**) studies. Adapted from Panta et al. (2016)

References

Absinta M, Ha SK, Nair G et al (2017) Human and nonhuman primate meninges harbor lymphatic vessels that can be visualized noninvasively by MRI. Elife. 6:e29738. https://doi.org/10.7554/eLife.29738.001

American Psychiatric Association (2013a) Diagnostic and statistical manual of mental disorders, 5th Edition (DSM-5). Diagnostic Stat Manual of Mental Disorder 4th Ed TR. 280. https://doi.org/10.1176/appi.books.9780890425596.744053

American Psychiatric Association (2013b) Highlights of changes from DSM-IV to DSM-5. Focus (Madison) 11(4):525–527. https://doi.org/10.1176/appi.focus.11.4.525

Andreasen NC, Nopoulos P, Magnotta V, Pierson R, Ziebell S, Ho B-C (2011) Progressive brain change in schizophrenia: a prospective longitudinal study of first-episode schizophrenia. Biol Psychiatry 70(7):672–679. https://doi.org/10.1016/j.biopsych.2011.05.017

Armanfard N, Reilly JP, Komeili M (2016a) Local feature selection for data classification. IEEE Trans Pattern Anal Mach Intell 38(6):1217–1227. https://doi.org/10.1109/TPAMI.2015.2478471

Armanfard N, Komeili M, Reilly JP, Mah R, Connolly JF (2016b) Automatic and continuous assessment of ERPs for mismatch negativity detection. In: Proceedings of the Annual International Conference of the IEEE Engineering in Medicine and Biology Society, EMBS, vol 2016. IEEE, Piscataway, pp 969–972. https://doi.org/10.1109/EMBC.2016.7590863

Armanfard N, Reilly JP, Komeili M (2017) Logistic localized modeling of the sample space for feature selection and classification. IEEE Trans Neural Networks Learn Syst 29(5):1396–1413. https://doi.org/10.1109/TNNLS.2017.2676101

Bellman RE, Dreyfus SE (1962) Applied dynamic programming. Ann Math Stat 33(2):719–726. https://doi.org/10.1289/ehp.1002206

Berk M, Conus P, Lucas N et al (2007) Setting the stage: from prodrome to treatment resistance in bipolar disorder. Bipolar Disord 9(7):671–678. https://doi.org/10.1111/j.1399-5618.2007.00484.x

Bishop CM (2006) Pattern recognition and machine learning. Springer, Berlin. https://doi.org/10.1117/1.2819119

Breiman L, Spector P (1992) Submodel selection and evaluation in regression. The X-random case. Int Stat Rev 60(3):291–319. https://doi.org/10.2307/1403680

Cao B, Passos IC, Mwangi B et al (2016) Hippocampal volume and verbal memory performance in late-stage bipolar disorder. J Psychiatr Res 73:102–107. https://doi.org/10.1016/j.jpsychires.2015.12.012

Cao B, Stanley JA, Passos IC et al (2017a) Elevated choline-containing compound levels in rapid cycling bipolar disorder. Neuropsychopharmacology 42(11):2252–2258. https://doi.org/10.1038/npp.2017.39

Cao B, Mwangi B, Passos IC et al (2017b) Lifespan gyrification trajectories of human brain in healthy individuals and patients with major psychiatric disorders. Sci Rep 7(1):511. https://doi.org/10.1038/s41598-017-00582-1

Cao B, Passos IC, Mwangi B et al (2017c) Hippocampal subfield volumes in mood disorders. Mol Psychiatry 22(9):1–7. https://doi.org/10.1038/mp.2016.262

Cao B, Luo Q, Fu Y et al (2018) Predicting individual responses to the electroconvulsive therapy with hippocampal subfield volumes in major depression disorder. Sci Rep 8(1):5434. https://doi.org/10.1038/s41598-018-23685-9

Chawla NV, Bowyer KW, Hall LO, Kegelmeyer WP (2002) SMOTE: synthetic minority over-sampling technique. J Artif Intell Res 16:321–357. https://doi.org/10.1613/jair.953

Colic S, Wither RG, Lang M, Zhang L, Eubanks JH, Bardakjian BL (2017) Prediction of antiepileptic drug treatment outcomes using machine learning. J Neural Eng 14(1):016002. https://doi.org/10.1088/1741-2560/14/1/016002

García-Laencina PJ, Sancho-Gómez J-L, Figueiras-Vidal AR (2010) Pattern classification with missing data: a review. Neural Comput Appl 19(2):263–282. https://doi.org/10.1007/s00521-009-0295-6

Hastie T, Tibshirani R, Friedman J (2009) The elements of statistical learning. Springer, New York. https://doi.org/10.1007/978-0-387-84858-7

Haukvik UK, Westlye LT, Mørch-Johnsen L et al (2015) In vivo hippocampal subfield volumes in schizophrenia and bipolar disorder. Biol Psychiatry 77(6):581–588. https://doi.org/10.1016/j.biopsych.2014.06.020

Haykin S (2009) Neural networks and learning machines, vol 3. Prentice Hall, Upper Saddle River doi:978-0131471399

He H, Garcia EA (2009) Learning from imbalanced data. IEEE Trans Knowl Data Eng 21(9):1263–1284. https://doi.org/10.1109/TKDE.2008.239

Kapczinski NS, Mwangi B, Cassidy RM et al (2016) Neuroprogression and illness trajectories in bipolar disorder. Expert Rev Neurother 7175:1744–8360 (Electronic):1–9. https://doi.org/10.1080/14737175.2017.1240615

Khodayari-Rostamabad A, Hasey GM, MacCrimmon DJ, Reilly JP, de Bruin H (2010) A pilot study to determine whether machine learning methodologies using pre-treatment electroencephalography can predict the symptomatic response to clozapine therapy. Clin Neurophysiol 121(12):1998–2006. https://doi.org/10.1016/j.clinph.2010.05.009

Khodayari-Rostamabad A, Reilly JP, Hasey GM, de Bruin H, MacCrimmon DJ (2013) A machine learning approach using EEG data to predict response to SSRI treatment for major depressive disorder. Clin Neurophysiol 124(10):1975–1985. https://doi.org/10.1016/j.clinph.2013.04.010

Kohavi R (1995) A study of cross-validation and bootstrap for accuracy estimation and model selection. IJCAI 14(2):1–7. https://doi.org/10.1067/mod.2000.109031

Le QV A tutorial on deep learning part 2: autoencoders, convolutional neural networks and recurrent neural networks. Google Brain. 2015:1–20

Le Roux N, Bengio Y (2008) Representational power of restricted Boltzmann machines and deep belief networks. Neural Comput 20(6):1631–1649. https://doi.org/10.1162/neco.2008.04-07-510

Müller KR, Mika S, Rätsch G, Tsuda K, Schölkopf B (2001) An introduction to kernel-based learning algorithms. IEEE Trans Neural Netw 12(2):181–201. https://doi.org/10.1109/72.914517

Panta SR, Wang R, Fries J et al (2016) A tool for interactive data visualization: application to over 10,000 brain imaging and phantom MRI data sets. Front Neuroinform 10:1–12. https://doi.org/10.3389/fninf.2016.00009

Passos IC, Mwangi B, Vieta E, Berk M, Kapczinski F (2016) Areas of controversy in neuroprogression in bipolar disorder. Acta Psychiatr Scand 134(2):91–103. https://doi.org/10.1111/acps.12581

Peng H, Long F, Ding C (2005) Feature selection based on mutual information: criteria of max-dependency, max-relevance, and min-redundancy. IEEE Trans Pattern Anal Mach Intell 27(8):1226–1238. https://doi.org/10.1109/TPAMI.2005.159

Rajkomar A, Oren E, Chen K et al (2018) Scalable and accurate deep learning for electronic health records. npj Digit Med 1(1):1–15. https://doi.org/10.1038/s41746-018-0029-1

Ravan M, Reilly JP, Trainor LJ, Khodayari-Rostamabad A (2011) A machine learning approach for distinguishing age of infants using auditory evoked potentials. Clin Neurophysiol 122(11):2139–2150. https://doi.org/10.1016/j.clinph.2011.04.002

Ravan M, MacCrimmon D, Hasey G, Reilly JP, Khodayari-Rostamabad A (2012) A machine learning approach using P300 responses to investigate effect of clozapine therapy. In: Proceedings of the Annual International Conference of the IEEE Engineering in Medicine and Biology Society, EMBS. IEEE, Piscataway, pp 5911–5914. https://doi.org/10.1109/EMBC.2012.6347339

Rumelhart DE, Hinton GE, Williams RJ (1986) Learning representations by back-propagating errors. Nature 323(6088):533. https://doi.org/10.1038/323533a0

Schapire RE (2003) The boosting approach to machine learning: an overview. Nonlinear Estim Classif 171:149–171 doi:10.1.1.24.5565

Soutullo C, Chang K (2005) Bipolar disorder in children and adolescents: international perspective on epidemiology and phenomenology. Bipolar Disord 7(6):497–506. http://onlinelibrary.wiley.com/doi/10.1111/j.1399-5618.2005.00262.x/full

Stein JL, Hibar DP, Madsen SK et al (2011) Discovery and replication of dopamine-related gene effects on caudate volume in young and elderly populations (N1198) using genome-wide search. Mol Psychiatry 16(9):927–937. https://doi.org/10.1038/mp.2011.32

Trautmann S, Rehm J, Wittchen H (2016) The economic costs of mental disorders. EMBO Rep 17(9):1245–1249. https://doi.org/10.15252/embr.201642951

Van Leemput K, Bakkour A, Benner T et al (2009) Automated segmentation of hippocampal subfields from ultra-high resolution in vivo MRI. Hippocampus 19(6):549–557. https://doi.org/10.1002/hipo.20615

Vigo D, Thornicroft G, Atun R (2016) Estimating the true global burden of mental illness. Lancet Psychiatry 3(2):171–178. https://doi.org/10.1016/S2215-0366(15)00505-2

Whiteford HA, Degenhardt L, Rehm J et al (2013) Global burden of disease attributable to mental and substance use disorders: findings from the Global Burden of Disease Study 2010. Lancet 382(9904):1575–1586. https://doi.org/10.1016/S0140-6736(13)61611-6

Williams EG, Auwerx J (2015) The convergence of systems and reductionist approaches in complex trait analysis. Cell 162(1):23–32. https://doi.org/10.1016/j.cell.2015.06.024

Woods KS, Doss CC, Bowyer KW, Solka JL, Priebe CE, Jr WPK (1993) Comparative evaluation of pattern recognition techniques for detection of microcalcifications in mammography. Int J Pattern Recognit Artif Intell 7(6):1417–1436

A Clinical Perspective on Big Data in Mental Health

3

John Torous, Nikan Namiri, and Matcheri Keshavan

While the word *analysis* holds special meaning in psychiatry from a psychodynamic therapy perspective, our lives are also constantly being analyzed by machines. Whether we realize it or not, computers have been fully integrated into our lives and devices, ranging from the smartphone we use for phone calls, the cars we use to drive, and the internet we use to communicate across. All of these computers contain algorithms that seek to analyze and understand our behaviors or intentions: the smartphone to remind of appointments and recommend navigation routes, the car to automatically brake if a child jumps in the road, the search engine to offer website links to answer a question. The same algorithms that make today's computers useful are not only restricted to increasing efficiency, ease, and comfort. They can also be, and already are, used to study, predict, and improve mental health. In this chapter we explore the rapidly expanding field of digital psychiatry with a focus on the synergy between data and algorithms that hold the potential to transform the mental health field.

As discussed in other chapters, the accessibility of new technologies, like smartphones, and access to the data they generate have paved new roads for innovation and discovery in many fields. Among them, mental health has received

J. Torous (✉)
Division of Digital Psychiatry, Beth Israel Deaconess Medical Center, Harvard Medical School, Boston, MA, USA

Department of Psychiatry, Beth Israel Deaconess Medical Center, Harvard Medical School, Boston, MA, USA
e-mail: jtorous@bidmc.harvard.edu

N. Namiri
Department of Bioengineering, University of California Los Angeles, Los Angeles, CA, USA

M. Keshavan
Department of Psychiatry, Beth Israel Deaconess Medical Center, Harvard Medical School, Boston, MA, USA

I. C. Passos et al., *Personalized Psychiatry*,
https://doi.org/10.1007/978-3-030-03553-2_3

some of the most prominent advances. Consider for a moment the vast amount of information a smartphone can provide relevant to behavior and mental health. Geolocation data can provide objective measures of exercise and activities, phone call and text message logs measurement of social engagement, voice samples clues to mood, error rates in typing a window into cognition and mental state, and so on. There is so much data generated from smartphones alone that there is a need for collaboration with data science fields in order to help make sense of these myriads. Understanding this collaboration and work, along with the intersection of psychiatry and data science, offers an exciting window into the new world of big data.

To understand this new world of data and algorithm, it is first necessary to lay a groundwork in the concepts of big data and machine learning. While these two terms are often used broadly and their exact definitions are beyond the scope of this chapter—understanding their meaning in the context of clinical psychiatry is an important first step.

Big data is characterized by three principles: velocity, volume, and variety, together known as the three V's of big data. Smartphones utilized for mental health offer an example of high velocity data, as data streams such as geolocation, keyboard strokes, and phone call logs are constantly flowing through from devices and into computers where the data can be stored. Smartphones in mental health are also a paradigm for high volume data, as smartphones can provide a constant data stream from features, such as accelerometer and CPU, which provide millions of data points in a matter hours. In addition to the velocity and volume, smartphones are an example of the variety in big data. Consider the wide range of data types a smartphone can collect that is relevant to mental health, ranging from geolocation to weather data, call and text logs to light sensors, voice data to keyboard strokes, and more. Thus, when considering the velocity, volume, and variety of smartphone data for mental health, it is easy to see why this big data is unlike most other data streams currently utilized in clinical psychiatry.

An issue arising from the mass quantities of big data is creating effective means of analyzing and drawing accurate conclusions from the data, which is precisely where machine learning comes in. Other primary issues include the ethics, patient perspective, security, and appropriate clinical utilization of this data, which are covered in the upcoming sections, as well as later chapters.

The analysis of these big datasets and further extrapolation into feasible application is the crux of machine learning. Machine learning enables physicians and researchers alike to analyze patient data using methods novel to the clinic. The nature of big data means that we need computers to assist in finding meaning or patterns in the data. This does not mean that a psychiatrist allows the computer to make clinical judgments, but rather that he/she allows the computer to suggest potentially useful information garnered from a sea of big data from, for example, a patient's smartphone. Perhaps the machine learning algorithm noted a pattern that when the patient does not leave the home or exercise, mood worsens. This is information the psychiatrist can now use to inquire more and start a discussion with the patient. To find these patterns in the data, the machine accesses mass amounts of data points and organizes them using statistical learning methods.

Statistical learning in machine learning consists of three major subsets: supervised, unsupervised, and semi-supervised learning.

Supervised learning requires a predetermined learning algorithm for the machine, which includes two essential parts: features and outcomes. The features (i.e. time spent at home), which are the predictors of the outcome (i.e. severity of depressive symptoms), are given to the machine as variables for it to then construct models for the most predictive outcomes.

Unsupervised learning, the second method, is similar to supervised learning in the sense that the machine is tasked with categorizing patients based on data. However, unsupervised learning does not possess programmed predictors; instead, the machine sifts through datasets in order to find its own parameters from which to then group patients. This process, known as clustering, requires the machine to perform dimensionality reduction, by which unlikely predictors are eliminated while the remaining ones are used to form relationships with patient outcomes. For example, no one may have programmed the computer to find a relationship between outgoing text messages and manic episodes through supervised learning, but in unsupervised learning the computer is able identify this unseen relationship. Of course many of these new relationships may not be useful in the clinic, as discussed later in this chapter. The psychiatrist must be wary that statistical significance is not the same as clinical significance.

The third and final type is semi-supervised learning, which combines the methods of supervised and unsupervised learning. In semi-supervised learning, only a small subset of the patients have a known outcome, and the rest of the patients are used to corroborate or change the initial relationship.

However, the brief above descriptions of machine learning and big data makes one critical assumption. In Desjardins the clinical world there is always missing or messy data. A patient may not recall how he reacted to a medication, may forget the name of his prior prescriber, is unsure if he was ever diagnosed with bipolar disorder, and so on. Likewise, big data itself is not perfect and often is messy and rife with missingness. Perhaps the geolocation sensor on the phone was not perfectly calibrated, turned off to save battery, or there was a mistake in the app recording that data. Thus prior to inputting into the machine, data may undergo cleaning, a process that removes subjects, or at least part of their data, from the dataset if their data is too messy or has too much missing. While superficially harmless, removing subjects from datasets has the potential to skew analysis, particularly if the removed subjects or data points are from the same group. Consider the simple example of patients with depression turning off their smartphone because they may not want to be contacted by others. This simple turning of an on/off switch means that no data is gathered and much is missing, when these data points could have provided valuable insight into the patient's symptoms.

As an alternative to cleaning messy data, missing data may be filled in through approximation using classical statistics, or statistical learning methods. The general linear regression model (GLM) is the simplest of statistical learning methods. GLM utilizes regression models to develop correlation coefficients between features and outcomes; however, this leads to the issue of overfitting in the case of high-dimensional datasets. Overfitting occurs when modeling of specific parameters fit too closely with a given dataset. Using a larger sample size combats this overfitting, by minimizing the effects of outliers and data that may be merely noise. Although increasing the volume of data will eliminate overfitting, the problem still lingers in high-dimensional research studies, in which the number of parameters is far greater than the number of observations.

Other techniques include elastic net models, a further extension of GLM, which use a large set of features to predict outcomes. Elastic nets will then filter through and select only the highest correlated predictors to incorporate into the final model. This is a manifestation of data reduction: the elimination of particular parameters in order to provide a highly correlated, accurate, and simplistic model for big datasets. Naïve-Bayes and Classification and Regression Trees (CART) are two additional methods of statistical learning. Naïve-Bayes is essentially an application of Bayes' Theorem, in that it classifies the likelihood of an event based on the value of one known variable. This variable is assumed to be independent of other parameters. CART, on the other hand, maps complex relationships between variables using a methodology similar to a flowchart. Data is first split up into categories, each represented as a leaf on the flowchart. The leaves are then connected to outcomes as well as other leaves, depending on the leaf's predictive capabilities.

Mental health research can produce significantly more powerful results when datasets from multiple sources are compiled into one and analyzed as a single dataset. Such analyses require large computational power, but are feasible, as demonstrated by several recent analysis into adolescent alcohol misuse for predicting current and future patterns (Whelan et al. 2014). In this study, an elastic net model was utilized to select for only the most impactful predictors of adolescent overconsumption. The resulting parameters included life experiences, neurobiological nuances, and overall personality of the adolescent. Moreover, the model provided regression values for each predictor, and based on these values, the model was able to remain accurate after application to a new data set. This dataset of new adolescents served to test the model, while the initial set of adolescents were used to first train and create the model. Typically, a dataset of K samples is subdivided, and all but one sample (K-1) is used to properly train and configure the model. Once the model is developed, the last sample is used for a test run, which hopefully results in a low prediction error. This process is repeated K times, each time resulting in a new set of K-1 subgroups for model training, while leaving the final subgroup for testing. This process is referred to as K-fold cross validation, and is widely utilized, including by studies presented later in this chapter.

3.1 Examples of Machine Learning Today in Psychiatry: Medication Selection

Despite tremendous recent increases in psychiatric knowledge of psychopharmacology, in today's world, finding the right medication for a patient can still be a process of trial and error. It can be hard to know a priori which patients will respond well to an antidepressant, and which may find the side effects too hard to bear or may simply not have an adequate response. While clinical experience is crucial in these decisions, machine learning offers both the patient and psychiatrist new information that may augment medication selection.

Matching the right antidepressant medication to the right patient is not trivial. Considering even a simplified definition of depression—meeting five of nine symptoms listed in the DSM-5 for 2 weeks—there are, in mathematical terms, nine choose five combinations of presenting symptoms, which is a total of 126. Biological evidence also suggests that there are subtypes of depression and that different types of depression respond better to certain medications than others. Machine learning can cluster patient symptoms into predictive subsets, from which psychiatrists can then prescribe the optimal prescriptions, targeted for a specific symptom within the patient's general depression.

The following examples (Chekroud et al. 2016, 2017) offers a model based on complete and prior collected data in the Sequenced Treatment Alternatives to Relieve Depression (STAR*D) trial, meaning the challenges of missingness and messiness are not addressed. This study used machine learning to create models to help identify whether a patient will benefit from a particular medication based entirely on the patient's unique background and clinical symptoms. Data from STAR*D (1949 usable patients) was used to construct a 25-predictor model to accurately estimate patient remission from the antidepressant citalopram, a serotonin reuptake inhibitor.

The three most predictive factors of non-remission were baseline depression severity (0.07793), restlessness during the last 7 days (0.06929), and lowered energy level over the last 7 days (0.05893). The most predictive characteristics for remission were having a job (−0.06946), years of education (−0.04712), and loss of insight of the depressive symptoms (−0.04625). The model was internally validated using the STAR*D dataset, resulting in an accuracy of 64.4%, higher in comparison to most predictive clinical models. The model was taken one step further and tried for validation on an external dataset, Combining Medications to Enhance Depression Outcomes (COMED). The COMED patient data was divided into three groups: escitalopram plus placebo, escitalopram plus buproprion, and venlafaxine plus mirtazapine. The predictive accuracy for each group was 59.6%, 59.7%, and 51.4%, respectively. Although the latter treatment group did not create statistically significant results ($p = 0.53$), the other two groups were significant, suggesting this model as promising for predicting medications that would best serve a patient.

The point of such a model is not to replace a psychiatrist, but rather to offer a new tool that may be useful in informed decision making regarding medication selection. Of course before any model can become widely adopted for clinical use, it also must be validated in real world conditions with real world data—which is often messy and missing to some degree. Such research efforts are currently underway and will continue to refine the field's knowledge about matching the right medication to the right patient. Chapter 4 will further discuss this topic.

3.2 Examples of Machine Learning Today in Psychiatry: Suicide Prediction

In the United States, suicide rates have risen to a 30 year high, tragically making suicide one of the top ten causes of death among those aged 10–64 (Curtin et al. 2016). Despite suicide awareness and outreach, this represents a 24% increase since 1999 (Tavernise 2016), and serves as an urgent call to action. While universal screening for suicide is a goal, it is not yet the standard, as implementation serves as the chief barrier. Patients and healthcare providers alike need a simple, yet effective means of quickly identifying risk factors for potential suicidal patients during preliminary evaluations. The grave disparity among research advances and current suicide rates has opened the door for machines learning and big data.

There is an urgent need for new tools to assist in predicting and preventing suicide. As alluded to above, while many area of health such as cancer and infectious diseases have experienced remarkable decreases in mortality rate as well as diagnostic and preventative advancements, suicide rates have increased. Current models to predict suicide risk have only little to moderate predictive utility, deeming previous suicidal attempts as the most common risk factor. Yet the fact that 60% of suicides are performed by those who have never made prior attempts reveals the weakness of these current models (Christensen et al. 2016).

New data and algorithms offer the potential to improve suicide prevention by extending monitoring beyond the clinic, with the ability to even respond to that data in real time. Interfacing with social media also provides machines a mechanism for identifying those at risk in real-time. In November 2017, Facebook announced it will be using artificial intelligence to monitor user's feeds in an attempt to predict who may be at risk (Zuckerberg 2017). While Facebook has not yet revealed what data they utilize and what algorithms they use, social media is becoming an active area of machine learning and mental health research. Other social media platforms are important targets as well for machine learning efforts. Machines can detect tweets and the changes within them that raise flags for suicide. However, further data mining must be performed in order to better characterize profiles of those at risk, and may soon include facial and voice characteristics as markers. By combining big data analysis by machines with individually gathered data streams, short-term risk factors can be quantified and identified almost immediately to provide needed support.

Medical records themselves also provide a source of data for machine learning techniques to offer new information relevant to suicide prevention. A case in point is a study from Montpellier University Hospital, where the records of 1009 hospitalized suicide attempters were analyzed in terms of several clinically-relevant parameters, including impulsiveness, mental disorders, and childhood trauma (Lopez-Castroman et al. 2016). This data was used for a hierarchical ascendant classification to create three homogeneous phenotypic clusters. The first cluster, labeled impulse ambivalent ($n = 604$), contained patients who were characterized by relatively non-lethal means of attempts and planning. The second cluster, well-planned ($n = 365$), had carefully planned attempts, more alcohol or drug abuse prior to the attempt, and had patients who employed more precautions to avoid interruptions. The third group, called frequent ($n = 40$), was the smallest, and included patients with more total attempts, being more serious and violent, and childhood abuse.

There were significant differences between each cluster for all analyzed variables ($p < 0.001$). Of the three clusters, clusters 1 and 2 were the most similar in terms of patient phenotype, so multivariate analysis with CART was performed on these two clusters. Cluster 3, on the other hand, was relatively distinct, possessing a female majority and a prevalent number of tobacco smokers, 90.0% and 80.6% of the cluster, respectively. This cluster was also prevalent in patients with anorexia nervosa (91.7%) and anxiety disorder (23.5%). Clustering is important as it offers clinically relevant and actionable insights that can be used to help clinicians identify those at high risk today. As more research continues, these models will continue to improve.

Clustering is not the only machine learning method useful for suicide prediction. Research groups across the world are actively investigating new data streams as well as new methods. For example, one group explored a neural network model for risk assessment of emergency room patients. The researchers created a software screening tool that 91% of patients found easy to complete, taking an average of 0:56 min, compared to nearly 8 min for a psychiatrist's brief evaluation (Desjardins et al. 2016). In preliminary testing, the neural network model was very accurate in predicting these new datasets, displaying a 91% accuracy in predicting psychiatrist's risk assessment and 89% for assessment of psychiatric intervention. This model provides the initial steps towards emulating the gold standard in evaluating suicide risk, but like all results, this model will need to be re-produced and run with new data to demonstrate its true clinical potential.

Related to suicide, non-suicidal self-injury (NSSI), most common among children and young adults, is deliberate self-injuring without suicidal intentions. The typical lifetime prevalence of NSSI in young adults and children is 13.9–21.4%, and the most common manifestation of NSSI is cutting (Plener et al. 2016). The internet is the most frequently used means by which NSSI health information is obtained. This information is sought not only by those who self-injure, but also the individuals who seek ways to help those who self-injure (*i.e.* parents and caregivers).

A recent study looked at the quality of the web resources for non-suicidal self-injury and highlighted the need for both mental health professionals and internet consumers to be cautious with what they read (Lewis et al. 2014). Researchers from the University of Guelph in Ontario, Canada searched 92 terms related to NSSI that resulted in 1000 Google hits or more. The first page of hits from these terms were evaluated, and the quality of health information on each website was evaluated using established guidelines from the Health On Net (HON) Foundation. They found that each of 340 healthcare websites contained an average of 1.44 ± 1.18 (mean $\pm$ SD) myths about NSSI. The most prominent myths were associating NSSI with a mental disorder (49.3%), abuse (40%), or that women are more likely to self-injure (37%). The mean quality of healthcare information in terms of HON criteria was 3.49 ± 1.40, while only one website received a perfect score of 7. Moreover, very few of these websites were credible, as only 9.6% were endorsed by health (*i.e.* hospitals) and/or academic institutes.

These results are concerning for not only patients but also machine learning efforts. Without proper collaborations between psychiatry and data science fields, it is easy to see how incorrect information could easily be accessed and programmed into machine learning algorithms. The advantage of machine learning tools is they can be delivered at scale to the population, but this is likewise their weakness, as incorrect or harmful information can be similarly scaled as well. Chapter 5 will further discuss this topic.

3.3 Examples of Machine Learning Today in Psychiatry: Symptom/Outcome Monitoring

Machine learning methods can do more than predict risk of self-harm or suicide; they can also help guide treatment decisions such as identifying the right medication for the right patient. For example, one third of patients suffering from Major Depressive Disorder (MDD) do not react adequately to treatment. Much effort has been put into characterizing treatment-resistant depression (TRD), defined as an inability to achieve at least 50% reduction in depression (McIntyre 2014). To investigate the potential of machine learning methods, 480 patients with TRD were studied to identify predictors for ineffective treatments (Kautzky et al. 2017). This patient cohort was taken from the Group for the Study of Resistant Depression (GSRD), a multinational European research consortium. A machine learning model was created using 48 predictors from clinical (change of sleep, suicidality), sociodemographic, and psychosocial (marital status, education) patient aspects. A Random Forest algorithm was used for model development, and results demonstrated that using all 48 predictors resulted in an accuracy of 73.7% for resistance and 85.0% for remission. However, single predictors resulted in an odds ratio of only 1.5; even the strongest single predictor, time between first and last depressive episodes, resulted in merely 56% and 60% accuracy for resistance and remission, respectively. Likewise, clinical predictions made by psychiatrists for treatment resistance are not dictated by a single parameter, but rather by considering many factors of the patient. The clinical line of thinking is reflected by this machine, in that more parameters create a better diagnosis, and may help optimize treatments in the clinic.

Machines do not need to rely solely on previously collected data, as they have demonstrated the ability to learn and make accurate predictions from real-time data. Ecological momentary assessment (EMA) is an important tool used by healthcare professionals to evaluate the mental state of patients throughout their daily activities. However, EMA has typically been administered through self-report questionnaires, leading to response bias and subjectivity. In this era of increasingly ubiquitous smartphones, EMA can be easily conducted via phone-based sensors and surveys, which are becoming more prevalent in psychiatry research. With their myriad of sensors, such as GPS, accelerometer, and ambient light, smartphones can provide real-time information about patient environment. The social logs of smartphones, such as call/text logs and social media profiles, also offer clues about social interactions and communication patterns (Torous et al. 2016).

A study by Asselbergs et al. offered new insights into mental health by demonstrating the potential of real-time phone data when combined with machine learning methods (Asselbergs et al. 2016). A mobile phone app was implemented on 27 Dutch university students to monitor their moods through proxies of social activity, physical activity, and general phone activity. The data was used for predictive modeling, including personalized predictive models for each participant based on individual data from their previous days. A regression algorithm selected and weighed variables into subsets to predict self-monitored mood. The eMate mobile app prompted subjects to evaluate their mood at five set points per day. Two-dimensional and one-dimensional mood evaluations were used, the latter of which simply asked the subject to rate his/her mood on a 10-point scale. The two-dimensional scale, however, used two levels of valence: positive and negative affect.

The unobtrusive, real-time data aspect for the study was collected using iYouVU, a faceless mobile app founded on Funf open-sensing framework. This app collects pre-determined sensor data and app logs, which are then sent over Wi-Fi to a central server. Daily averages of EMA, both one and two-dimensional, were averaged and scaled to each subject. The unobtrusive data included total number of times screen was turned on/off, and call and SMS text message frequency to top five contacts.

The personalized mood prediction machines for each student were created using forward stepwise regression (FSR), in which relevant variables for predicting mood are selected sequentially as more data is accumulated. To maximize predictive variables while avoiding overfitting, only eight variables (the number of data points (42) divided by 5) were used in each student's model. The first FSR was stepAIC procedure, which selects variables based on Akaike information criteria (Akaike 1974). The second FSR method was stepCV procedure, by which variables are selected based on their ability to lower cross-validated mean square error between the phone-collected scores and cross-validated predicted scores. Thus a variable is added to the model unless it increases the mean squared error. The cross validation was performed using leave-one-out cross validation (LOOCV) by predicting residual sum of squares for every model run. The predictive performance of both FSR variants was evaluated using LOOCV, comparing the observed mood rating through the mobile phone with that predicted by the personalized FSR models. The result were relatively underwhelming, as the proportion of correct predictions was 55–76% lower compared to two previously published naive models. This result demonstrates that machine learning methods are not always better than simple baseline models.

However, sometimes machine learning does produce results that are not seen with simpler models or clinical observations alone. A case in point is a study involving speech data and schizophrenia (Bedi et al. 2015). Disorganized speech is often an early sign of prodromal schizophrenia, and a novel study analyzed speech data with machine learning in order to accurately predict schizophrenia conversion among youths with prodromal symptoms. Utilizing latent semantic analysis (LSA), an algorithm that utilizes multiple dimensions of associative analysis of semantic speech structure, researchers studied speech data for over 2.5 years in those at risk for becoming schizophrenic. LSA assumes that the meaning of a word is based on its relation to every other word in the language; words that recur together many times in a transcript can then be indexed in terms of their semantic similarity. A machine learning algorithm was trained using the semantic vectors generated from LSA from those who developed psychosis (CHR+) and those who did not (CHR-) upon follow-up. The machine used a cross-validated classifier, analogous to *K*-fold cross validation, to learn the speech features which differentiated CHR+ from CHR- participants. Results demonstrated 100% accuracy in predicting psychosis for each participant within the sample used to generate the machine. Not surprisingly, this perfect result is significantly greater than the predictive capability of clinical classifiers from the SIPS/SOPS evaluation (79%). However, the machine was not externally validated on a new dataset different from the initial one used for model fabrication. The true predictive capability of the model is likely lower than the apparent perfect accuracy. Although, automated analysis clearly demonstrates the potential to outperform standard clinical ratings for predicting clinical onset, as machines can provide insight on minute semantic difference that the latter cannot sense.

3.4 Next Step and the Future of Machine Learning in Psychiatry

3.4.1 Outsource Simple Tasks to Machines

While machine learning will not replace psychiatrists, it can help make their work more efficient. Machines have the ability to fully automate generic tasks within psychiatry, such as symptom severity screening. At the time of this writing, The National Health Service in the United Kingdom is assessing an artificial intelligence app, developed by the company Babylon, on nearly 1.2 million users in London, England (Burgess 2017). Rather than have citizens call the non-emergency health service phone line, which is typically understaffed and run by non-medically trained individuals, the app provides a promising alternative through a virtual physician evaluation. This app possesses a database of symptoms which is utilized by the app's chatbot to help patients instantly find out the urgency of their health issues. When presented with a serious case, as assessed by the machine, the chatbot connects patients directly to a physician. The app has demonstrated the ability to assess patient illness in a more accurate manner than phone line operators, while also saving government resources.

3.4.2 Population Level Risk Stratification and New Disease Models

Machine learning methods can also help psychiatry with population level risk prediction. Mental health disorders are typically predicted with machines using single time point cross-sectional variables, most often clinical aspects from initial evaluations. These machines may be compromised by their inability to account for the dynamic nature of symptoms. Thus, predictive modeling can benefit by assessing the micro-level (momentarily/daily) and macro-level (monthly/yearly) dynamic factors that impact the course of psychiatric illnesses (Nelson et al. 2017).

The same models can also offer new ways to conceptualize disease. Dynamic Systems Theory proposes that complex systems consist of sub-systems that are interconnected and highly correlative, while other sub-systems possess diverse aspects that are only loosely related. Distinguishing the sub-systems that are correlative has provided a means for researchers to accurately model aspects of mental illness, one of which is through the EMA. As previously mentioned, this assessment evaluates an individual's mood at many points in a day to detect shifts from baseline. Such micro-level assessment lends to correlations between depressive symptoms and subtle changes in emotional state. On the other hand, recording macro-level changes is done through joint modeling of event outcomes and time-dependent predictors.

These complex systems are also the crux of Network Theory. By using Network Theory, we assume mental disorders are a result of complex relationships between the biological, psychological, and social aspect of our lives. Each system is triggered by the other, resulting in an overall system that is characterized by positive feedback, forming a type of loop, whereby the body may be stuck in a continuous cycle of particular symptoms. These symptoms can sometimes be malicious, which can then be classified as states of mental disorder. Similarly, Instability Mechanisms convey that mental disorders are the result of amplifying minor health issues by feedback loops in the body. What initially seems like a commonplace affect, such as disliking of cramped rooms, can exacerbate into claustrophobia for some individuals if the body is continuously running the loops.

3.4.3 Better Use of Medical Records Data

Machine learning can help not only in better characterizing psychiatric illness, but also in improving the delivery of psychiatric care. Though clinical assessment remains the paradigm for patients seeking diagnosis, there is increasing interest in using retrospective patient records as big datasets. Retrospective data has gained popularity due to its ability to simplify and standardize medicine for more precise results. Electronic health records (EHRs) provide a means of retrospectively phenotyping patients, and correlating their characteristics, whether demographic or diagnostic, to treatment outcomes. But using EHR data can be difficult and combining EHR data across multiple clinics and health systems is a serious challenge due to lack of interoperability. The *green button* movement seeks to make it easier to operationalize EHR data and utilize it in novel ways, such as to learn how a particular patient may respond to treatment compared to others with a similar presentation (Longhurst et al. 2014). This process of screening EHRs was used to change the conventional policy for setting alarm alert limits, which is typically age-based. Lucile Packard Children's Hospital of Stanford operationalized 1000 of EHRs to create a novel distribution of alarm limits for children, based on their heart rate distribution rather than age. This nascent implementation of personalized database data has helped provide more accurate care tailored for each of the pediatric patients.

Physicians have also begun to take initiative in promoting collaboration between researchers in the digital health field through secure sharing of health records and data. Dr. Ashish Atreja, Chief Technology Officer at Icahn School of Medicine at Mount Sinai, has facilitated digital health data sharing among physicians through the digital platform NODE Health (Comstock 2017). This initiative allows for secure sharing of clinical data in efforts of providing a wide range of researchers with patient data that would otherwise be unattainable for them. The researchers who take part in NODE Health are able to foster multi-site projects, rather than conduct costly duplicate studies, because the data is readily available for sharing.

3.5 What are the Next Steps to Realize that Future

3.5.1 A Need for High Quality Data

Despite the early successes and continued promises of machine learning methods for mental health, there is also need for caution. One area regards bias that may inadvertently be scaled up by these methods if the wrong types of data are used to build models. For example, collecting and processing information through social media poses a challenge, as the information is highly skewed by search methods. There have been few studies that address search filters, combinations of keywords and search rules, in their entirety. In a similar vein, very few research groups provide the proportion of usable data that is collected by their filters. Bias in search filters can skew data, which precludes generalizable results. The proportion of quality data that results from search filters must be objectified and characterized in relation to a standard benchmark. Such a benchmark has been aimed to be created by a recent study, which aimed to provide standards for retrieval precision and recall (Kim et al. 2016)

Twitter, for example, is one of the most prevalent social media platforms used to gather data, largely in part due to its high volume. When obtaining data from Twitter, researchers must be aware of colloquial slang, abbreviated words (due to the limit on characters per Tweet), and use of hashtags. Experts in the field of study should be utilized for assistance in filter selection. Signal to noise ratio is also imperative and keywords with a low ratio should be excluded. This threshold ratio depends on the study, but one benchmark to discard tweets is those that result in less than ten tweets in a month or return less than 30% of relevant tweets. The search rules can use Boolean operators, such as AND, NOT, OR, as well as data pre-processing techniques like n-grams and proximity operators.

3.5.2 A Need for Good and (New) Study Design

New tools like machine learning may also require new clinical study designs to make the most efficient use of the resulting data. Ensuring that studies are designed to have not only appropriate controls but also appropriate training and testing datasets must be considered when seeking to utilize supervised machine learning methods. When aiming to utilize unstructured methods, it is useful to consider how data may cluster and whether the outcome metric is suitable. Close partnerships with data scientists are critical to ensure that statistical methods are employed correctly and that spurious correlations or findings are avoided (Ioannidis 2016). Health studies can also learn from the software paradigm of agile development, in that iterative and rapid studies may prove of more value to single long studies that are committed to one particular technology or method. This concept, sometimes referred to as Agile Science, offers an early roadmap of a new way to envision and execute clinical studies (Hekler et al. 2016)

3.5.3 A Need to Realize and Plan for Unintended Consequence

Though machine learning demonstrates the ability to improve the medical field through means such as increased predictive accuracy, there are also unintended side effects. When novel technologies are introduced to healthcare, some aspects of medicine can suffer. One major concern is the over reliance on machine learning to detect symptoms and proposed treatments for patients. This can lead to deskilling, decline in performance when a task becomes automated, which can result in drastic deficits if the technology is removed. Mammogram readers, for example, experienced a 14% decrease in sensing diagnostic markers on images with computer-aided detection (Cabitza et al. 2017).

It is also difficult to fully program machines to consider the clinical parameters that may be only detectable by a holistic, human evaluation. The human experience can sense psychological, social, and relational issues, aspects which must then be quantitatively programmed into data that is interpretable by a machine. Evidently, the problem lies in coding these subtle characteristics that only the human senses are conditioned to perceive. This also encompasses fundamental guidelines of healthcare, which can be overlooked in machines because they are merely taught to recognize patterns in data. For example, a risk prediction machine was created for 14,199 patients with pneumonia, and the machine found that those with both asthma and pneumonia had a lower mortality risk than patients solely with pneumonia (Cabitza et al. 2017). Clinicians were surprised that asthma could be a protective agent, and began questioning the legitimacy of the machine. However, the clinicians could not find a problem with the machine, as it had merely done its job as it had been programmed to do. The issue lied in the coded parameters and data. Patients with both asthma and pneumonia were assigned to intensive care units, which resulted in a 50% reduction in mortality risk than patients with solely pneumonia, who were typically not admitted to intensive care. Contextual factors such as the difference in hospital unit are crucial for accurate modeling, though are difficult to recognize and then accurately encode into machines.

3.6 Conclusion

The future is bright for machine learning in mental health. In recent years, researchers have published numerous studies showing the potential of these methods for predicting suicide, matching patients to the right medicine, increasing efficiency of care, and even monitoring patients outside of the hospital with smartphones and sensors. However, it is worth noting that much of this research has yet to be reproduced or deployed at scale in healthcare systems. Given the nascence of machine learning applied towards mental health, compounded by the challenge of quantifying human behavior, it is not surprising that the field is still exploring its role and potential. But given the direct errors as well as unintended consequences, a cautious approach is warranted. Nonetheless, as the diverse methods and applications of this chapter underscores, the field is rapidly progressing and we expect the impact and role of machine learning in mental health to only continue to grow.

References

Akaike H (1974) A new look at the statistical model identification. IEEE Trans Autom Control 19(6):716–723

Asselbergs J et al (2016) Mobile phone-based unobtrusive ecological momentary assessment of day-to-day mood: an explorative study. J Med Internet Res 18(3):e72

Bedi G et al (2015) Automated analysis of free speech predicts psychosis onset in high-risk youths. NPJ Schizophrenia 1(1):15030

Burgess M (2017) The NHS is trialling an AI chatbot to answer your medical questions. Wired. Available at http://www.wired.co.uk/article/babylon-nhs-chatbot-app/

Cabitza F et al (2017) Unintended consequences of machine learning in medicine. JAMA 318(6):517–518

Curtin S et al (2016) Increase in suicide in the United States, 1999–2014. National Center for Health Statistics, Hyattsville Brief No. 241. Available online at https://www.cdc.gov/nchs/products/databriefs/db241.htm

Chekroud AM et al (2016) Cross-trial prediction of treatment outcome in depression: a machine learning approach. Lancet Psychiatry 3(3):243–250

Chekroud AM et al (2017) Reevaluating the efficacy and predictability of antidepressant treatments: a symptom clustering approach. JAMA Psychiat 74(4):370–378

Christensen H et al (2016) Changing the direction of suicide prevention research: a necessity for true population impact. JAMA Psychiat 73(5):435–436

Comstock J (2017) Mount Sinai launches data sharing initiative for digital health pilots. MobiHealthNews, Portland Available at http://mobihealthnews.com/content/mount-sinai-launches-data-sharing-initiative-digital-health-pilots
Desjardins I et al (2016) Suicide risk assessment in hospitals: an expert system-based triage tool. J Clin Psychiatry 77(7):e874–e882
Hekler EB et al (2016) Agile science: creating useful products for behavior change in the real world. Transl Behav Med 6(2):317–328
Ioannidis JP (2016) Why most clinical research is not useful. PLoS Med 13(6):e1002049
Kautzky A et al (2017) A new prediction model for evaluating treatment-resistant depression. J Clin Psychiatry 78(2):215–222
Kim Y et al (2016) Garbage in, garbage out: data collection, quality assessment and reporting standards for social media data use in health research, infodemiology and digital disease detection. J Med Internet Res 18(2):e41
Lewis SP et al (2014) Googling self-injury: the state of health information obtained through online searches for self-injury. JAMA Pediatr 168(5):443–449
Longhurst C et al (2014) A 'green button' for using aggregate patient data at the point of care. Health Aff 33(7):1229–1235
Lopez-Castroman J et al (2016) Clustering suicide attempters: impulsive-ambivalent, well-planned, or frequent. J Clin Psychiatry 77(6):e711–e718
McIntyre RS (2014) Treatment-resistant depression: definitions, review of the evidence, and algorithmic approach. J Affect Disord 156:1–7
Nelson B et al (2017) Moving from static to dynamic models of the onset of mental disorder: a review. JAMA Psychiat 74(5):528–534
Plener PL et al (2016) The prevalence of nonsuicidal self-injury (NSSI) in a representative sample of the German population. BMC Psychiatry 16(1):353
Whelan R et al (2014) Neuropsychosocial profiles of current and future adolescent alcohol misusers. Nature 512(7513):185
Tavernise S (2016) US suicide rate surges to a 30-year high. New York Times, New York. Available online at http://www.nytimes.com/2016/04/22/health/us-suicide-rate-surges-to-a-30-year-high.html?_r=0
Torous J et al (2016) New tools for new research in psychiatry: a scalable and customizable platform to empower data driven smartphone research. JMIR Mental Health 3(2):e16
Zuckerberg M (2017) Here's a good use of AI: helping prevent. Suicide. Available online at https://www.facebook.com/zuck/posts/10104242660091961

Big Data Guided Interventions: Predicting Treatment Response

4

Alexander Kautzky, Rupert Lanzenberger, and Siegfried Kasper

4.1 Introduction

While big data and advanced statistics have been on the rise all across science and start to slowly ingress everyday life, they have just in recent years found their way into neuropsychiatric research (Passos et al. 2016). The exponentially increasing amounts of both, data generation and availability, have paved the way for the advance of data driven analytical approaches, labeled by the term statistical learning. Psychiatry may especially stand to benefit from these trends as a lack of biomarkers for almost all of the major disorders as well as corresponding treatment options has troubled psychiatrists for almost half a century. Despite endeavors to determine clinical, genetic, epigenetic as well as imaging risk factors or treatment moderators, progress on defining clinically relevant predictors for treatment of psychiatric disorders on the individual level has so far been marginal.

Thereby, affective disorders and the most common major depressive disorder (MDD) may be particularly afflicted with these issues. While increasing prevalence rates due to social developments or tightened awareness have been reported for MDD for years, our knowledge concerning the biological scaffoldings of the disorder is still shaky. In fact, most of the research on MDD has traditionally adopted a binary approach, comparing single clinical, sociodemographic or genetic features in MDD patients to controls or between different treatment outcome phenotypes. Even though a plethora of studies have carved out convincing evidence for many predictors of MDD or treatment outcome, their actual diagnostic and predictive worth for an individual patient has been underwhelming. Therefore, implementation of multivariate models, usually adopting so-called advanced statistics with

A. Kautzky · R. Lanzenberger · S. Kasper (✉)
Medical University of Vienna, Department for Psychiatry and Psychotherapy, Vienna, Austria
e-mail: alexander.kautzky@meduniwien.ac.at; sci-genpsy@meduniwien.ac.at

I. C. Passos et al., *Personalized Psychiatry*,
https://doi.org/10.1007/978-3-030-03553-2_4

supervised or unsupervised learning capacity, has been advised by almost all recent reviews on the topic (Perlis 2016; Cohen and Derubeis 2018).

MDD has been a primary target of machine learning approaches within the last 10 years and the etiological, diagnostic and clinical pitfalls of the disorder make it a suitable target to reconsider advances and shortcomings of statistics and big data in psychiatry. In the following chapter, supervised and unsupervised learning techniques aimed to predict treatment outcome for antidepressants in MDD will be discussed, exemplary for big data guided interventions in psychiatry.

MDD ranks among the most frequent diseases worldwide, showing a lifetime prevalence of about 20%. Between 3% and 3.8% of global disability adjusted life years in 2010 were caused by MDD, making it the fourth leading cause of estimated global disease burden (WHO 2001). The goal of precision medicine in MDD, allowing prediction of treatment outcome on the individual patient level, may require optimization of the various predictors already at hand rather than searching for a new biomarker. The urgency of this ambition may best be understood considering that 30–60% of MDD patients do not show sufficient symptom remission after the first antidepressant agent was administered. An estimated 15% remain significantly ill even after multiple treatment algorithms, thus considered to be affected by treatment resistant depression (TRD) (Thase 2008). All treatment approaches are time consuming and consequently about a fifth of patients are still severely disabled by their disease 2 years after treatment initiation. Consequently, the identification of risk factors and reliable predictors for treatment outcome has become a medical but also socioeconomic issue.

4.2 Depressive Subtypes: Unsupervised Learning Techniques in MDD

MDD may be the clinically most diversely presented neuropsychiatric disorder. The diagnostic requirements for MDD according to ICD-10 and DSM V allow high heterogeneity and several competing symptom severity scores like Hamilton depression rating scale (HAM-D), Montgomery-Åsberg depression rating scale (MADRS), Quick inventory of depressive symptomatology (QIDS) or Becks depression inventory (BDI) are in clinical use, often applied concurrently. There are over 50 different symptoms referenced by the most popular depression rating scales and several hundred unique combinations of depressive symptoms all lead to the same diagnosis. Oftentimes obverse symptoms like appetite and sleep de- or increase lead to similar total scores. Accordingly, recent literature has emphasized the lack of reproducibility between different rating scores for MDD (Fried et al. 2016; Fried 2017). Along these lines, heterogeneity within MDD has been proposed and definition of subgroups of patients with distinct features may facilitate better treatment algorithms.

The idea of depressive sub-types is by no means new and traditionally melancholic and atypical depression have been highlighted in research. DSM V just recently adopted the anxious subtype of depression. Conventional approaches usually define different subtypes first and compare these by means of different variables and treatment effects. For example, in a large German multicenter study comprising over 1000 MDD patients, melancholic subtypes showed a higher rate of early symptom improvement under antidepressant (AD) treatment while anxious and atypical MDD showed worse treatment outcome (Musil et al. 2018). On the other hand, another large European multicenter study showed worse treatment outcome for melancholic depression (Souery et al. 2007). While these studies have produced interesting results, the inconsistence of the findings and small effect sizes for the respective subtypes rendered the prognostic value for treatment outcome insufficient (Arnow et al. 2015).

Advanced statistics allow a different approach to this dilemma by unsupervised learning techniques as k-means, hierarchical clustering or latent class analysis (LCA). Thereby, subtypes are not predefined by clinical observations but recognized in a data-driven way. An exhaustive review of data driven subtypes in MDD from 2012 showed on one hand a lack of such studies, and on the other hand the failure to reproduce stable data-driven subtypes in multiple samples up to that point (Van Loo et al. 2012). Investigations were hindered by several factors, including insufficient or divergent information regarding MDD symptoms captured by the severity rating scores, differences in baseline severity and treatment effects. Based on these findings, the conventional approach of defining subtypes just by depressive symptoms was mostly abandoned for a broader scope featuring also sex, comorbidities and other clinical data.

Based on these earlier studies, in the last years unsupervised machine learning produced some seminal results in MDD. Van Loo et al. could demonstrate that specific symptom clusters rather than total severity scores were predictive of long term treatment outcome in MDD (Van Loo et al. 2014). Exploiting the large database of the WHO Surveys, including over 8000 respondents to AD treatment, they defined a cluster by the k-means algorithm featuring high degree of suicidality, anxiety symptoms as irritability and panic, and early disease onset that was predictive of longer hospitalization, chronic MDD as well as higher disability and severity. The high-risk cluster thereby comprised up to 70% of adverse outcome. Comparing the k-means clustering results to generalized linear model (GLM) results, they could also demonstrate the advantages of stratification by symptom clusters rather than conventional multivariate models. A follow-up analysis also implemented comorbidities and could increase the prognostic value of the clusters, predominantly driven by anxiety disorders (Wardenaar et al. 2014).

In concordance with these findings, another study using the Netherlands Mental Health Survey with over 1300 MDD patients registered highlighted four clusters defined by severity and comorbid anxiety that showed distinctive clinical characteristics and treatment outcome, including use of mental health services and long-term disability (Ten Have et al. 2016).

The Sequenced Treatment Alternatives to Relieve Depression (STAR*D) sample was also screened for data-driven MDD subtypes with machine learning techniques. Ulbricht et al. surfaced four clusters within baseline data of over 2000 MDD patients receiving Citalopram, defined by severity, insomnia and increased appetite

(Ulbricht et al. 2015). Thereby, clinical and outcome characteristics varied between clusters and sex differences were suggested. Women were significantly more likely to be within the increased appetite cluster but showed slightly better response rates than men within the same cluster. Interestingly, in follow-up analyses focusing on cluster transition after 12 weeks of treatment, they could show divergent trajectories for men and women (Ulbricht et al. 2016, 2018). While male MDD patients were clustered according to severity and psychomotor agitation or slowing, female patients were clustered by severity and appetite change. Severely depressed patients were naturally less likely to achieve symptom resolution, but interestingly, predominantly psychomotor agitation for men and decreased appetite for women defined the least likelihood for remission.

The studies described above have surfaced a spectrum of data-driven subtypes based either on diagnostic symptoms alone or a broader range of clinical and sociodemographic predictors. There are few communalities, except for clustering according to baseline severity and comorbidities as anxiety disorders or symptoms, and none of these sub-types were reliably reproduced in other data sets than those in which they were generated. Their actual predictive power remains therefore undetermined. Considering the differences in data registration, e.g. inclusion criteria and consequently baseline severity, applied diagnostic and severity assessment tools or outcome measures, a final answer to the existence and characterization of depressive subtypes will probably not even be provided by advanced statistics in the near future.

However, while data-driven studies are still lacking concision, they have also shown consistency in their results. Some predictors as anxiety symptoms showed high agreement within all analyses and consequently, the idea of trans-diagnostic, symptom-based subtypes beyond MDD got traction in the last years. Based on the often overlapping symptoms of affective disorders, Grisanzio et al. studied data deriving from the Brain Research and Integrative Neuroscience Network Foundation including approximately 200 patients with either MDD, panic disorder or posttraumatic stress disorder as well as 200 healthy controls. Applying hierarchical clustering to this data set revealed six clusters defined by tension, anxious arousal, general anxiety, anhedonia, melancholia and normative mood (Grisanzio et al. 2018). Despite the rather small sample size, clusters spanned over all three diagnoses and could be replicated in an independent sample collected by the same group at Stanford University. Following the idea of big data, the group also implemented multimodal predictors as electroencephalography-recorded β power and functional capacity scores that provide further classification.

Interestingly, also another study in a large cohort of 73,000 subjects, deemed representative for the general adult population of the northern Netherlands, could demonstrate clusters of depression and anxiety symptoms independently of diagnosis of affective disorders (Wanders et al. 2016). Thereby, especially a cluster of clinically relevant symptoms showed significant overlap and was related to disability.

In summary, most data-driven studies on definition of depressive subtypes did not support the conventional classification of anxious, atypical and melancholic depression. Findings advocate a role of anxious symptoms that may impact subtypes in a transdiagnostic fashion and even characterizes subclinical populations. These results endorse the use of extensive, quantitative and translational symptom assessment as proposed by research domain criteria (RDoC) and neuroscience-based nomenclature (NbN). While unsupervised data-driven approaches have already brought neuropsychiatric research one step closer to the goal of precision medicine, their future success will be dependent on

(a) the precision of the applied diagnostics and symptom assessment tools, preferably using rescaleable quantitative scores rather than binary questions, and overcoming flaws like the same coding for opposite effects (e.g. weight gain or decrease, hypo- or hypersomnia)
(b) interoperability of data sets to allow consequent validation
(c) implementation of multimodal data, including clinical, sociodemographic, genetic, epigenetic and imaging data and
(d) refinement of statistical techniques, probably combining unsupervised learning with other machine learning tools.

Some of the studies described above already used a combination of unsupervised and supervised machine learning for variable selection for clustering. This design was also chosen by a study within the data pool of the "Group for the Study of Resistant Depression" (GSRD), applying RandomForest (RF) for interaction-based variable selection and subsequently k-means clustering to surface subgroups of patients with distinct response trajectories to AD (Kautzky et al. 2015). At its time, this was the first study to combine genetic and clinical parameters for prediction of treatment outcome in TRD, aimed at risk stratification for patients receiving antidepressant therapy by identification of parsimonious signatures of variables. RF identified four out of 20 genetic and clinical predictors selected based on earlier single factor association studies to be most informative. These were SNPs within *HTR2A*, *BDNF*, and *PPP3CC* genes and melancholic depression. k-means clustering further characterized a risk phenotype based on these predictors, indicating higher chances of responding to therapy in a subgroup of patients without melancholic depression and carrying homozygotes of the T allele of rs6313 of the *HTR2A* gene, of the G allele of rs6265 of the *BDNF* gene as well as of the rs7430 polymorphism of the *PPP3CC* gene. This signature increased the odds to respond to antidepressant therapy 4-times compared to patients without this specific combination. The opposite signature might be associated with TRD, however, still be irrelevant for the clinical routine as none of the patients comprised in that sample featured this combination. Still, melancholic patients lacking the putatively protecting homozygote G alleles of rs6265 and rs7430 as well as homozygote T alleles of rs6313 showed an increased rate of treatment resistance of 83% compared to 66% in the whole sample (Table 4.1).

However, the main goal of statistical learning algorithms has traditionally been prediction of treatment outcome on individual patient level.

Table 4.1 Studies introducing data-driven subtypes for major depressive disorder (MDD)

Study	Sample	Algorithm	Clusters subtypes	Features	Predictive for	Validation
van Loo et al. (2014)	8261 WMH	k-means	3	Suicidality, anxiety symptoms, early disease onset	Hospitalization, chronic MDD, disability, severity	No
Wardenaar et al. (2014)	8261 WMH	k-means	3	van Loo et al. (2014) + fear, distress and externalizing disorders	Hospitalization, chronic MDD, disability, severity	No
Ten Have et al. (2016)	1388 NMHS	LCA	4	Severity and anxiety	Psychiatric service use, long-term disability	No
Ulbricht et al. (2015)	2772 STAR*D	LCA	4	Severity, increased appetite, insomnia	PTSD, GAD, bulimia, social phobia, remission	No
Ulbricht et al. (2016)	755 STAR*D	LCA	4	Severity and appetite	Treatment response	No
Ulbricht et al. (2018)	387 STAR*D	LCA	4	Severity and psychomotor symptoms	Treatment response	No
Grisanzio et al. (2018)	420 INNFD	HC	6	Tension, anxious arousal, general anxiety, anhedonia, melancholia, mood	Behavioral and physiological functioning	External
Kautzky et al. (2015)	225 GSRD	k-means	5	Melancholia, rs6313 of *HTR2A*, rs6265 of *BDNF*, rs7430 of *PPP3CC*	Treatment response	No
Chekroud et al. (2017)	STAR*D	HC	3	HAM-D symptom clustering: core emotionlal, atypical, sleep	Treatment response (AD specific)	External

Sample sizes, the algorithms used for clustering or definition of latent variables, number of clusters, the most distinctive clinical and sociodemographic features and predictive qualities are reported

WMH world mental health surveys, *NIHM* Netherlands mental health survey, *STAR**D* sequenced treatment alternatives to relieve depression, *INNFD* integrated neuroscience network foundation database, *GSRD* group for the studies of resistant depression, *LCA* latent class analysis, *HC* hierarchical clustering

4.3 Prediction of Treatment Outcome

While simple classification tools like logistic regression have long been staples in psychiatric research, they produced overall disappointing and sometimes conflicting results even in big data sets (Carvalho et al. 2014). This might be owed to the heterogeneous and complex symptomatology of the phenotype TRD that represents a decisive clinical but also methodological challenge. A major obstacle is the lack of a generally accepted definition for TRD despite extensive discussions about criteria and staging systems since the first scientific description by Heimann and colleagues back in 1974 (Thase 2008). Thus, several TRD definitions are currently coexisting, deviating in dosage, duration as well as number of AD trials required for treatment resistance. In addition, outcome criteria like the severity scores applied or thresholds used for response and resistance vary widely between studies. Thus, even the most embracing definition of TRD, characterized by a score indicating severe affection on a recognized symptom severity scale after application of at least one AD treatment algorithm of adequate dosage and duration, may show differences between studies and data sets, making comparability difficult. According to most definitions, however, at least two failed AD trials must be applied to reach TRD, allowing even more room for variation. For some staging systems, classes of AD treatments are considered hierarchically, requiring selective serotonin reuptake inhibitors (SSRIs), tricyclic antidepressants (TCA), monoaminoxidase A (MAO) inhibitors and electro-convulsive therapy (ECT) for different stages of treatment resistance respectively (Dold and Kasper 2016; Schosser et al. 2012).

4.3.1 Big Data: Sociodemographic, Clinical and Genetic Predictors

Considering the small effect sizes expected for single predictors for TRD, mostly multicentered, multinational research groups have contributed to the definition of reliable sociodemographic, clinical and genetic markers of treatment outcome. Prominent examples would be the European research consortium GSRD or the US-American STAR*D trial (Sinyor et al. 2010; Schosser et al. 2012). The largest study in TRD at its time, conducted by Souery et al. (2007), could link comorbid panic disorder and social phobia, comorbid personality disorder, suicidal risk, high symptom severity, melancholic features, more than one previous hospitalization, recurrent major depressive episodes (MDE), non-response to the first administered AD and age of onset before turning 19 to TRD (Souery et al. 2007). Other studies could replicate these findings and also associated long duration and high severity of the current MDE, outpatient status, high suicidal risk, MDD in first or second degree relatives, longer hospitalization over lifetime, comorbid panic disorder, melancholic and psychotic features and the occurrence of adverse effects during the treatment with TRD (Balestri et al. 2016). Considering sociodemographic predictors, a higher risk of TRD in patients with a demanding, high occupational level was shown as well as for unemployed patients and those with low educational degree (Mandelli et al. 2016). Somatic comorbidities have sometimes been studied to no definite conclusion.

In addition to those psychosocial and clinical predictors, there is evidence for the fundamental importance of genetics in MDD. Twin studies proved a high heritability of about 40%, but the contribution of a specific genetic variant to the etiology of MDD and outcome of AD treatment is still speculated upon and may explain less than 0.05% of heritability (Sullivan et al. 2000). On the other hand, an estimated variance in treatment outcome of 42% explained by all common variants together has been implied (Tansey et al. 2013). Hence, a plethora of interacting SNPs and epigenetic mechanisms can be expected to shape the pathophysiology of MDD rather than distinct polymorphic variations (Gratten et al. 2014). Over the last decade, several candidate-gene as well as genome wide association studies (GWAS) have been conducted in MDD with regards to treatment outcome. Investigations performed by the GSRD and other groups associated SNPs from several candidate genes involved with the serotonergic system with TRD, among them *COMT*, *CREB1*, *BDNF*, *5HTR1A* and *5HTR2A*, *GRIK4*, *GNB3* and *PPP3CC* (Schosser et al. 2012; Perlis et al. 2009, 2010). An abundance of candidate gene studies was performed, resulting in a synopsis of hardly comprehensible findings and lack of replication. Negative and inconsistent results may be owed to insufficient statistical power or disregard of epigenetic effects as methylation or gene-gene interactions. To address the first problem and to enable an unconcealed look at the genetics of MDD, several GWAS have been presented since 2010. Usually requiring far superior numbers than candidate gene approaches, multi-site research consortia like STAR*D, GSRD, the international SSRI Pharmacogenomics Consortium (ISPC), Genome-Based Therapeutic Drugs for Depression (GENDEP), combining medications to enhance depression outcomes (COMED) or Antidepressant Medication Pharmacogenomics Study (PGRN-AMPS) with sometimes several dozen thousands of MDD cases paved the way for GWAS in depression. First negative results for genome-wide associations with MDD were followed up in increasingly big cohorts and different stratification tactics, e.g. by gender, age or MDD subgroups, to compensate higher heterogeneity in MDD compared to other neuropsychiatric disorders like schizophrenia. Nevertheless, GWAS data on AD response, especially addressing specific ADs, is still limited and collected in distinctively smaller samples, mostly comprising a few hundred to thousand patients. So far, GWAS did not yield clinically relevant findings for predicting treatment outcome in MDD (Biernacka et al. 2015; Jung et al. 2017; Tansey et al. 2012). While an earlier study of the GENDEP project presented an association of rs2500535 within the uronyl 2-sulphotransferase gene with Nortriptyline response, most studies reported negative results on the genome wide level (Uher et al. 2010). For example, a study performed for examination of genetic contributors to duloxetine response in 391 MDD patients failed to produce any genome wide associations for drug response (Maciukiewicz et al. 2017).

As a putative remedy to small single marker effects, polygenic risk scores (PGS), adding up single marker effects identified in GWAS and validating them in independent samples to get a hold of their predictive quality, were introduced and anticipated to expedite new drug targets and precision medicine (Breen et al. 2016). Indeed, PGS could successfully be applied to some disorders as schizophrenia (Vassos et al. 2017). However, PGS underperformed in prediction of treatment outcome in MDD. A large study exploiting the GENDEP and STAR*D datasets could not find PGS predictive for AD response in over 2000 patients, however, lead to the conclusion that genetic risk for a disorder may not overlap with that for unfavorable treatment outcome (Garcia-Gonzalez et al. 2017). Interestingly, a recent study in the ISPC and PGRN-AMPS data sets predicting treatment response with consideration of personality traits yielded more positive results, with some associations within genes linked to *CRHR1* and *YEATS4*, which had previously been implicated in AD treatment outcome (Amare et al. 2018). The failure of GWAS and PGS may thereby be owed to the simple statistics, rather broadening conventional single factor analyses without fully capturing epistasis as well as psychosocial and clinical interaction effects. Consequently, big genetic data sets collected for GWAS were handled with advanced statistics to enable clinically relevant prediction for treatment outcome.

4.3.2 Supervised Learning Techniques in MDD: Towards Precision Medicine

Single factor approaches using conventional statistics consistently highlighted the involvement of clinical as well as genetic factors in TRD. Nevertheless, considered individually none of these predictors prove sufficient for detecting individuals at risk of resisting AD treatment (Gratten et al. 2014). Accordingly, recent reviews, e.g. by the think-tank of the Collegium Internationale Neuro-Psychopharmacologicum, have suggested focusing on a combination of predictors for diagnosis and treatment outcome of psychiatric disorders (Scarr et al. 2015). Just in recent years such models seem increasingly viable due to international efforts on data availability and intrusion of advanced statistics in psychiatry (Chen et al. 2011; Kennedy et al. 2012).

In the last decade more advanced statistical learning algorithms like regularized regression (elastic net, LASSO), support vector machines (SVM) or (RF) have been introduced as strategies for prediction of treatment outcome. Nevertheless, guidelines for selecting the most effective out of the already extensive repertoire of AD agents and strategies for subgroups or individual patients have not yet been established.

4.3.2.1 Supervised Learning Techniques in MDD: Clinical Predictors

Early adaptions of machine learning in prediction of treatment outcome were constrained by insufficient observation counts and fulfilled an exploratory role, showing advantages over conventional multivariate models without breakthrough and far from clinical application. For example, Serretti et al. compared logistic regression to neuronal network learning algorithms, yielding an accuracy of around 0.6 for treatment response to fluvoxamine in both, conventional and advanced statistical models (Serretti et al. 2007). However, several predictors neglected by the generalized linear model were considered by the machine learning approach, indicating better registration of interaction-based effects. Another study in a large cohort of over 1000 naturalistic MDD cases conducted by Riedel et al. again applied logistic regression, reaching a marginally better accuracy with six clinical predictors. Baseline severity scores, suicidality and psychotic features were consistently highlighted as the most important predictors in these studies, however, sometimes different directions were reported (Riedel et al. 2011). The authors also implemented regression tress, providing singular tree based hierarchical pathways, but still no significant improvement for prediction on a clinical level could be achieved.

The first somewhat successful endeavor of supervised learning techniques in predicting antidepressant treatment outcome was undergone by Perlis et al. (2013). Based solely on self-report questionnaire items, the authors presented a simple classification model featuring 15 selected variables that consistently reached an accuracy around 0.7 across training, test and validation sets comprised of STAR*D patients. A mixture of clinical predictors as QIDS self-rating items, including insomnia, energy and total score, as well as number of episodes and psychotic features, psychosociodemographic variables as gender, ethnicity and education, comorbidities as PTSD, and items hinting at environment interactions like trauma, showed the best discriminative properties. All these variables showed rather small odds ratios, hovering between 0.7 and 1.4, when considered separately. Intriguingly, in this study logistic regression proved on par accuracy but better stability compared to more sophisticated approaches as SVM, RF or Bayesian models. This might be owed to the wrapper-based selection algorithms preimposed on the training data, as variable selection based on importance for classification results is a main advantage of machine learning techniques as RF.

The selected predictors in these studies may not be surprising as they mostly agree with single factor results. The most significant risk factor in Perlis et al. turned out to be baseline QIDS total score, proving again that more severe cases are doing worse in treatment, even though a few studies suggested a more complex picture (Riedel et al. 2011). However, for the first time a ready-made prediction algorithm for an individual patient, possibly refinable for clinical use, was presented. Similar approaches were undergone within the GSRD data pool. A machine learning prediction model in using RF both for variable selection and classification of TRD and remission yielded again an accuracy above 0.7, indicating clinical significance (Kautzky et al. 2017a). This analysis was focused on sociodemographic and clinical predictors and, similar to Perlis et al., roughly 50 variables were included. Contrary to the earlier study, here the full set of 48 available predictors resulted in the maximum accuracy of 0.73 for resistance and 0.85 for remission, while a reduced set of the 15 most important predictors selected by RF importance measurement resulted in an accuracy of 0.62 for resistance and 0.78 for remission. Considerable limitations were the cross-sectional nature of the study and the lack of an independent validation set. Treatment outcome was determined only by a threshold on a single HAM-D score. Cross-validation was performed only in the training set for variable selection and a single cast on an internal test set split off the data for model generation was used for validation.

On the other hand, these results were followed up with a comparable endeavor in a new sample of 552 patients (Kautzky et al. 2017b). Similar prediction results were achieved, reaching an accuracy of 0.75 and a positive and negative predictive value of 0.80 and 0.68, respectively. Again, a strained set of 15 easily predictors that could be extracted within 10 min of clinical interview was tested and still yielded an accuracy above 0.7. However, due to some design differences between the two samples, including treatment outcome phenotypes TRD and response determined by change in MADRS scores over treatment and exact variable characterization as well as exclusion criteria, no cross-sample validation was performed.

Taken together, no definite conclusion on the most effective variable selection and prediction algorithms can be drawn yet. Nevertheless, these studies affirmed that combinations of predictors are clearly superior to single factors and some variables have consistently been highlighted as more informative. Furthermore, anticipation of failed treatment response would allow for a tighter protocol with earlier application of augmentation therapies or ECT. Nevertheless, none of these studies approached the sought-after rationale for selecting the appropriate out of apparently equal AD options beyond consideration of side effects (Bauer et al. 2015).

DeRubeis et al. tried to answer that question with a generalized linear model for prediction of HAM-D after either psychotherapy or antidepressant drugs in a sample of roughly 250 patients (Derubeis et al. 2014). They predicted two hypothetical HAM-D outcome values based on baseline HAM-D, predefined clinical variables and a dummy treatment variable and compared these to actual outcome scores of the longitudinal study data. However, the results were rather unsatisfactory. The standard error was around 7 points in HAM-D and the mean differences of predicted HAM-D between treatment arms surprisingly low, only making a meaningful clinical difference (assumed at a threshold of 3 points in HAM-D score) in 60% of the observations within the sample.

Thriving on the auspices of the earlier studies, Iniesta et al. first presented a prediction model based roughly 800 patients and clinical variables that generated and compared prediction models for specific AD drugs, in that case Escitalopram and Nortriptyline (Iniesta et al. 2016). In a computationally exhaustive design with elastic net regression in a cross-validation and permutation testing approach, they refined a set of demographic and clinical predictors out of 125 variables within the categories demographic data, baseline severity, depression subtypes, symptoms, and dimensions, stressful life events and medication history, to be most discriminative for treatment outcome. The yield was an area under the curve (AUC) of 0.72 for remission in the escitalopram set. These results are comparable to Perlis et al. and overall show agreement with some earlier single factor results concerning the selected variables. However, the crucial finding of this work was that different sets of predictors were superior for Escitalopram and Nortriptyline, respectively. The accuracy decreased decisively for the whole data set to reach beyond chance level classification for cross-drug prediction. Overall, depressed mood, reduced interest, decreased activity, indecisiveness, pessimism and anxiety were the most prominent predictors for symptom improvement, while body mass index, appetite, interest-activity symptom dimension and anxious-somatizing depression subtype were most informative for predicting remission.

The predictors contributing most to the respective models computed in the described studies showed some variation that can partly be explained by design differences. For example, age of first administration of an AD and the respective response as well as baseline depression rating scale showed the strongest impact on classification results in some studies but could not be implemented in others (Kautzky et al. 2017a, b). Comorbidities PTSD and social phobia showed relevance in some studies but were underrepresented in others. On the other hand, predictors corresponding to symptom severity, suicidality and recurrent MDD were associated to treatment outcome in almost all relevant studies.

Interestingly, the strongest results in the GSRD studies were obtained when using all available features, 47 and 48 sociodemographic and clinical variables, respectively (Kautzky et al. 2017a, b). Still, the predictive power was condensed within the most informative variables and RF may be more robust to overfitting than other machine learning techniques as elastic net regression, which may explain the different conclusion drawn by Perlis et al. and Iniesta et al., that careful selection of variables increases classification performance (Iniesta et al. 2016; Perlis 2013). Most of the roughly 50 clinical predictors, featured with some level of variation in all three of the respective studies, contributed little to the outcome and did reflect earlier single factor effects. However, the latter was also true for some of the high scoring predictors, indicating that interaction-based analyses produce divergent results from conventional statistics.

Similarly, some limitations are shared among these studies. Even though high reliability of machine learning algorithms as RF or regularized regression was suggested for data bases with sufficiently large observation counts, the actual relevance of a model can only be validated in an external data set. Although overall conformable prediction quality across these studies and mostly commendable management of training and test samples via cross-validation add liability to the results, none of these earlier studies implemented independent validation sets. Also, hardly any of these studies featured a full nested cross-validation design for feature selection and tuning of parameters. Hence, it is impossible to rule out false positive findings that have only value in the confinements of the samples they were derived from.

An expedient validation of the prediction models across big data sets like GSRD, STAR*D or GENDEP may be hindered by different definitions of treatment outcome phenotypes and parameter recording. For example, different characterization of treatment response phenotypes by introducing a baseline severity score and switching from MADRS to HAM-D in the younger sample impedes comparative analyses across the two independent GSRD data sets.

Furthermore, only few data sets provide longitudinal clinical evaluation. With some notable exceptions like STAR*D, for many studies only cutoffs for dosage and duration of AD treatment were standardized and patients were receiving the full range of AD agents as well as augmentation with mood stabilizers and antipsychotics, sometimes even ECT. For example, the majority of patients enrolled in the GSRD studies were receiving more than one AD. Only more stringent protocols like Iniesta et al. adopted in their approach allow clear stratification by antidepressant agent without fragmentation in subgroups too small for meaningful interpretation (Iniesta et al. 2016) (Table 4.2).

4.3.2.2 Multimodal Data: Combining Clinical, Genetic and Imaging Predictors

As described above substantial progress in prediction of treatment response could be achieved with clinical and sociodemographic predictors, but overall prediction performance was still underwhelming. Only few studies were able to implement data from imaging techniques and genetic findings in a multimodal approach true to the idea of big data. First advances described above made clear that confinement to a set of few candidate predictors will not lead to the desired prediction performance (Kautzky et al. 2015).

The first study to incorporate genome wide genetic data into a machine learning model was conducted by Maciukiewicz et al. (2018). They applied a commendable nested cross-validation design with inner loops for regularized regression for variable selection and hyperparameter tuning for SVM, and outer loops for model validation. However, the predictive power was underwhelming with an accuracy of below 0.6. Still, different genetic markers were identified as most informative compared to conventional GWAS conducted by the same group earlier (Maciukiewicz et al. 2017).

More promising results were produced by a follow up study by Iniesta et al. Genome wide genetic variants were added to sociodemographic and clinical variables to enhance the prediction quality of their earlier model (Iniesta et al. 2018). Compared to their first approach, a smaller portion of little over 400 patients was available for model generation and validation. Comparing again predictors for Nortriptyline and Escitalopram, different signatures of 20 variables were surfaced for each respective AD. Interestingly, mostly genetic predictors were selected by a stern variable selection algorithm and again, different results to single association results yielded in a GWAS analysis in the same sample were observed.

Concerning imaging biomarkers, earlier studies successfully deployed electroencephalography (EEG) to predict remission after AD treatment with various drugs (Caudill et al. 2015; Hunter et al. 2011). The term AD treatment response index was labelled, accounting for changes in EEG signal after one week of treatment. Considering the substantially longer average time for treatment response, this prediction may be useful despite its obvious flaw, being based on markers that can only be assessed after treatment was initiated.

With the advance of imaging techniques as magnet resonance imaging (MRI) and positron emission tomography (PET) in psychiatry, prediction of treatment outcome based on structural and functional neuroanatomical patterns showed obvious appeal. However, acquisition of such data is still distinctively more resource intensive than clinical or genetic data. As a consequence, data sets for imaging-based prediction

Table 4.2 Results for machine learning prediction of treatment outcome phenotypes for major depressive disorder (MDD)

Study	Sample	Predictors (n)	Feature selection	Best predictors	Algorithm	Sensitivity & specificity	Validation	Acc./AUC/SE/r
Serretti et al. (2007)	116	Clinical (15)	Expert	Severity, duration, suicidality, education, PSD	LR ANN	n.r.	Split data	Acc: 0.62
Riedel et al. (2011)	1014 GFWS	Clinical (24)	LR	*Response*: Duration, Suicidality, Baseline HAMD, Neuroticism, Hospitalizations *Remission*: Duration, b. HAMD, Hospitalizations, SomaticS.	LR CART	n.r.	CV	AUC: 0.62–68
Perlis (2013)	2555 STAR*D	Clinical (48)	Expert & LR	No. of MDE, psychotic symp., sex, race, b. QIDS, PTSD, marital status, education, trauma, QIDS insomnia & energy	LR	0.91, 0.26	CV	AUC: 0.72
Kautzky et al. (2017a)	480 GSRD	Clinical (48)	RF	Timespan 1st to last MDE, age at and resp. to 1st AD, suicidality, No. of MDE, panic disorder, patient status, education, thyroid disorders, diabetes	RF	0.63, 0.80	Split data	Acc: 0.73
Kautzky et al. (2017b)	GSRD	Clinical (48)	RF	Baseline MADRS, SIRS score, timespan 1st to last MDE, severity, education, profession, suicidality, age, BMI, No. of MDE, hospitalizations	RF	0.82, 0.63	CV	Acc: 0.75
DeRubeis et al. (2014)	250	Clinical (9)	Expert	No. of prior AD, No. of life stressors, PSD, employment, relationship status, IQ, chronic subtype, b. HAMD, age	LR	n.r.	CV	SE: 6.2 HAMD
Iniesta et al. (2016)	793 GENDEP	Clinical (125)	RR	*Escitalopram*: Indecisiveness, interest, preoccupation w. death, depressed mood, problems w. close people, fatigue, phobia, insomnia, anxiety	RR	0.62, 0.69	CV with repeats	AUC: 0.72

Iniesta et al. (2018)	430 GENDEP	Clinical (125) Genetic (524871)	RR	*Escitalopram:* appetite, sleep, SomaticS., interest, b. HAMD, fatigue + 9 SNPs *Nortryptiline:* 20 SNPs	RR	0.69, 0.71	Nested CV	AUC: 0.77
Chekroud et al. (2016)	4706 STAR*D COMED	Clinical (164)	LR	25 clinical predictors	GBM	n.r.	CV + External	Acc: 0.60
Chekroud et al. (2017)	7221 STAR*D COMED	Clinical (164)	LR	Different sets of 25 clinical predictors chosen for each prediction model for three data-driven subtypes of MDD	GBM	n.r.	CV + External	r: 0.04–0.36
Kautzky et al. (2015)	299 GSRD	Clinical (8) Genetic (12)	Expert + RF	Melancholia, rs6313 of HTR2A, rs6265 of BDNF, rs7430 of PPP3CC	RF	0.25, 0.84	Split data	Acc: 0.62
Maciukiewic et al. (2018)	183 LUNDBECK	Genetic (GWAS)	LR + RR	*19 SNPs:* rs2036270, rs7037011, rsll38545, rsll07372, rslll36977, rsll581838, rsll843926, rsl347866, rsl6932062, rsl999223, rs2710664, rs39185, rs4S20243, rs4685865, rs4777522, rs4954764, rs60230255, rs6550948, rs972016	SVM	0.58, 0.46	Nested CV	Acc: 0.52

Sample sizes, the algorithms used for prediction, number of variables and set of the most distinctive clinical and sociodemographic features as well as sensitivity, specificity and accuracy are reported

GFWS German framework study, *STAR*D* sequenced treatment alternatives to relieve depression, *GSRD* group for the studies of resistant depression, *GENDEP* genome-based therapeutic drugs for depression, *COMED* combining medications to enhance depression outcomes, *RF* RandomForest, *RR* regularized regression, *LR* logistic regression, *ANN* artificial neuronal networks, *CART* classification and regression tree, *SVM* support vector machines, *CV* cross-validation of AD response were exponentially smaller, usually consisting of a few dozen observations. Along these lines, none of the respective studies featured independent validation and stratification for specific antidepressants could not be performed yet. Earlier studies all featured SVM after feature reduction and leave-one-out cross-validation and reported accuracies ranging from approximately 0.7 to 0.8 (Marquand et al. 2008; Liu et al. 2012; Costafreda et al. 2009; Nouretdinov et al. 2011). Keeping in mind the low observation count and lack of validations sets, the reported accuracies rivaling or surpassing those of large studies on clinical and genetic predictors suggest potential, but also caution.

Two more recent studies flavored MRI imaging data with clinical parameters. Patel et al. reported high accuracy of almost 0.9 in predicting treatment outcome to various AD in late life depression in 33 patients (Patel et al. 2015). Interestingly, clinical predictors did not seem to improve prediction quality for treatment response but only for classification of patients versus controls. Only diffusion tensor imaging (DTI) and functional connectivity MRI markers were comprised in the optimal among several hand-picked feature sets for an alternating decision tree model, that outperformed several other algorithms including SVM and regularized regression. The second study featured the largest data set among MRI prediction studies for treatment outcome so far with roughly 120 observations (Schmaal et al. 2015). Three outcome phenotypes simplified here as remission, response and chronic MDD were characterized based on 2-year follow up data and classification with a technique similar to SVM and leave-one-out cross-validation. No automated feature selection algorithm was used but different combinations of clinical, functional and structural MRI data were compared. Only classification of remission versus chronic MDD trajectories was successful with over 0.7 accuracy featuring only emotional faces functional MRI data (Table 4.3).

Up to this point, no study has combined imaging, genetic and clinical data in a single statistical model. Epigenetic effects as methylation, which bear potential to disentangle inconsistencies reported for most candidate and GWAS studies on genetic predictors, have been completely neglected so far. Incorporation of these different data modalities may be key to the future success of prediction of antidepressant treatment outcome.

4.3.2.3 Combining Supervised and Unsupervised Learning: Dealing with Heterogeneity

The studies discussed earlier show that identification of multimodal predictors for specific therapeutic agents instead of general predictors for TRD will be necessary to advance machine learning prediction to the clinical routine. To deal with the exuberant amount of heterogeneity in MDD, probably combinations of different statistical learning approaches will have to be deployed in increasingly large datasets that can deal with stratification by various subgroups and treatment trajectories. An elaborate example of combined usage of unsupervised and supervised machine learning is the project published by Chekroud et al. in 2016–2017 (Chekroud et al. 2016, 2017). Exploiting the large data mines of STAR*D, CO-MED and a set of trials on duloxetine, they first established a prediction model based on

Table 4.3 Results for machine learning prediction of treatment outcome phenotypes for major depressive disorder (MDD)

Study	Sample	Predictors	Feature selection	Best predictors	Algorithm	Sensitivity & specificity	Validation	Acc./AUC
Marquand et al. (2008)	20	fMRI	No	3-back task	SVM	0.85, 0.52	CV	Acc: 0.7
Liu et al. (2012)	35	SMRI	PCA	Grey matter in frontal lobe, parietal lobe, temporal lobe, occipital lobe and cerebellum	SVM	n.r.	CV	Acc: 0.83
Costafreda et al. (2009)	37	sMRI	ANOVA	*Remisson:* rostral aCC, pCC, middle frontal gyrus, occipital cortex *TRD:* orbitofrontal cortex, superior frontal cortex, hippocampus	SVM	0.89, 08.9	CV	Acc: 0.89
Nouretdinov et al. (2011)	17	SMRI	t-test	aCC, pCC, orbitofrontal cortex	SVM	0.79, 0.79	CV	Acc: 0.79
Patel et al. (2015)	33	Clinical fMRI	Expert	Only fMRI markers (DTI & functional connectivity)	ADT	n.r.	CV	Acc: 0.89
Schmaal et al. (2015)	118	Clinical fMRI	No	Emotional faces task and clinical predictors	SVM	0.80, 0.67	CV	Acc: 0.69–0.73

Sample sizes, the algorithms used for prediction, number of variables and set of the most distinctive imaging features as well as sensitivity, specificity and accuracy are reported

fMRI functional magnet resonance imaging, *sMRI* structural magnet resonance imaging, *PCA* principal component analysis, *SVM* support vector machines, *ADT* alternating decision trees, *CV* cross-validation variable selection with regularized regression and gradient boosting machine that showed modest accuracy around 0.6. Intriguingly, again different feature selection and performance were reported for specific ADs, here Escitalopram compared to Mirtazapine and Venlafaxine. In a subsequent study, they could allocate baseline symptoms of two different severity scales HAM-D and QIDS to three clusters based on over 4600 observations. Contrary two other clustering approaches, they did not strive for identification of subtypes but applied hierarchical clustering of baseline score items to generate a set of more practical outcome measures that might better capture differences between AD. While earlier clustering and factor analyses suggested 3–5 symptom clusters with some consistency, they reflected neither data driven nor clinically based subtypes of MDD and were not featured for prediction of treatment outcome before (Shafer 2006). Ceckroud et al. suggested three clusters labelled as "sleep", "atypical" and "core emotional" and looked at conventional regression as well as machine learning prediction models in each cluster separately. Unsurprisingly, baseline scores of the respective clusters were the strongest predictor in each model, however, some predictors like sex for "atypical" or baseline total score for "core emotional" showed strong contribution only to specific clusters. Most importantly, different trajectories for ADs were reported for each cluster with clinically relevant variation of symptom improvement. Prediction accuracy increased after refinement by unsupervised learning compared to their first report. These findings contrast underwhelming results in extensive studies referencing the whole symptom severity score for treatment outcome that did find hardly any indications for preferences for specific ADs (Cipriani et al. 2018). Overall, more than 7000 cases from three independent multicenter projects add cogency to these results while exemplifying the high standards for precision medicine on the drug- and patient-specific level. Nevertheless, the prediction performance was still insufficient for practical application, even with a handy link allowing real time assessment of patients based on 25 clinical parameters provided by the authors.

4.4 Summary and Outlook

In summary, prediction models for TRD, response and remission consistently reached accuracies around 0.70 in MDD. While everyday clinical application requires higher predictive performance with accuracies beyond 0.8 and balanced sensitivity and specificity, these models were clearly superior to expert predictions and could further be refined by multimodal data from epigenetics or imaging tools as EEG or MRI. Easily obtainable sociodemographic and clinical predictors that can be explored within minutes at any referral center could already substantially facilitate the prospective assessment of treatment outcome and most recent results suggested even further stratification by combining genetic and clinical predictors. The lack of extern validation, being the putatively most relevant concern to machine learning models so far, may be overcome by the trends of open-use algorithms and shared data sets.

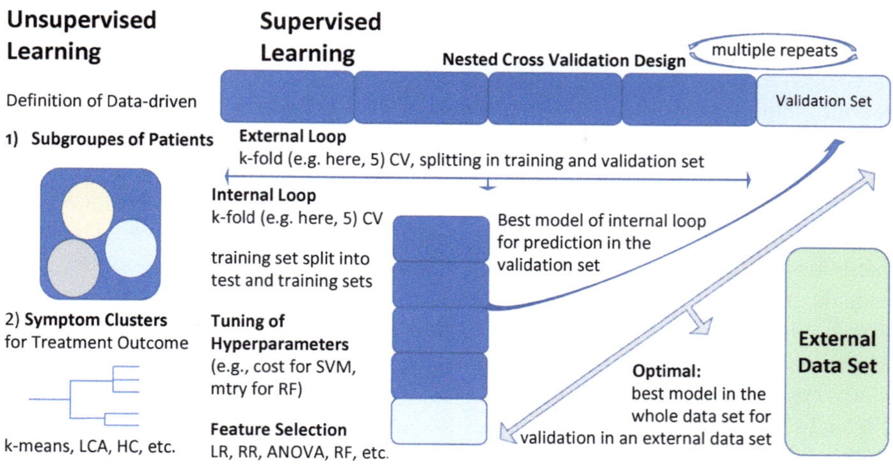

Fig. 4.1 Optimal modelling for advanced statistics for prediction of treatment outcome in major depressive disorder (MDD). First, stratification of patient subgroups may be performed with clustering or latent class analyses. Alternatively to conventional binary outcome measures or total score reduction, data-driven definitions of outcome measures may be computed with clustering. For prediction of treatment outcome, a nested cross-validation loop is recommended. The inner loop deals with hyperparameter tuning and feature selection while the outer loop is for model validation. Averages of accuracies retained over the outer loops should be reported, preferably after several repeats of the whole nested cross-validation. Permutation testing should be applied to test for significance. For optimal model validation, an external independent data set is necessary. *LCA* latent class analysis, *HC* hierarchical clustering, *RF* RandomForest, *RR* regularized regression, *LR* logistic regression, *SVM* support vector machines, *CV* cross-validation

Still, there is "no free lunch" in model generation for big data and advanced statistics in neuropsychiatry. Currently, different more and less conventional or advanced statistical learning algorithms are on par in prediction performance, including generalized linear models, regularized regression, neuronal networks, SVM and RF. As it seems unlikely that a specific algorithm will outclass the others across the board, thoughtful selection based on the data set at hand as well as comparative application will be required. To best adjust to heterogeneity and looseness in definition of symptoms and outcomes in MDD, a combination of unsupervised and supervised learning techniques may be the best choice. On the other hand, when depending only on data driven approaches, generalizability may be questionable and validation even more essential. As more and increasingly intricate models are required for capturing multiple outcome dimensions and stratification for different ADs or patients' subgroups at the same time, rigorous handling of quality measures like accurate variable selection, nested cross-validation or permutation testing will be key. To facilitate the implementation of these criteria, more generalizable symptom, severity and outcome definitions possibly beyond boundaries of ICD or DSM diagnoses, e.g. by adopting NbN and RDoC criteria, may be necessary.

Intriguingly, no studies have been conducted that implement machine learning models in a prospective way. Several ready-use models based on large data sets have been made public and a multi-step approach would be viable to test machine learning algorithms based on a first phase of data collection. Adopting AD trials based on prediction results at baseline could clearly demonstrate the clinical benefit of advanced statistics. The general information if a patient is likely to respond to AD agents would already allow for a faster administration of augmentation therapies or more invasive measures as ECT. Specific trajectories for ADs could facilitate choices for the first AD to be administered. Considering the existing models based on thousands of patients show accuracies already surpassing the threshold of clinical relevance, such studies could be planned even at these early stages of precision medicine in psychiatry. For a schematic depiction of an ideal study applying advanced statistics for prediction of treatment outcome please see Fig. 4.1.

Summarizing the findings of all relevant investigations for the most chatoyant disorder MDD, we believe that the scope to demonstrate the advantages of advanced statistics in neuropsychiatric research was met as the progression of results within the last years allows optimism for the goal of precision medicine on an individual patient level in mental health.

References

Amare AT, Schubert KO, Tekola-Ayele F, Hsu YH, Sangkuhl K, Jenkins G, Whaley RM, Barman P, Batzler A, Altman RB, Arolt V, Brockmoller J, Chen CH, Domschke K, Hall-Flavin DK, Hong CJ, Illi A, Ji Y, Kampman O, Kinoshita T, Leinonen E, Liou YJ, Mushiroda T, Nonen S, Skime MK, Wang L, Kato M, Liu YL, Praphanphoj V, Stingl JC, Bobo WV, Tsai SJ, Kubo M, Klein TE, Weinshilboum RM, Biernacka JM, Baune BT (2018) Association of the polygenic scores for personality traits and response to selective serotonin reuptake inhibitors in patients with major depressive disorder. Front Psych 9:65

Arnow BA, Blasey C, Williams LM, Palmer DM, Rekshan W, Schatzberg AF, Etkin A, Kulkarni J, Luther JF, Rush AJ (2015) Depression subtypes in predicting antidepressant response: a report from the iSPOT-D trial. Am J Psychiatry 172:743–750

Balestri M, Calati R, Souery D, Kautzky A, Kasper S, Montgomery S, Zohar J, Mendlewicz J, Serretti A (2016) Socio-demographic and clinical predictors of treatment resistant depression: a prospective European multicenter study. J Affect Disord 189:224–232

Bauer M, Severus E, Kohler S, Whybrow PC, Angst J, Moller HJ, WFSBP Task Force on Treatment Guidelines for Unipolar Depressive Disorders (2015) World Federation of Societies of Biological Psychiatry (WFSBP) guidelines for biological treatment of unipolar depressive disorders. Part 2: maintenance treatment of major depressive disorder-update 2015. World J Biol Psychiatry 16:76–95

Biernacka JM, Sangkuhl K, Jenkins G, Whaley RM, Barman P, Batzler A, Altman RB, Arolt V, Brockmoller J, Chen CH, Domschke K, Hall-Flavin DK, Hong CJ, Illi A, Ji Y, Kampman O, Kinoshita T, Leinonen E, Liou YJ, Mushiroda T, Nonen S, Skime MK, Wang L, Baune BT, Kato M, Liu YL, Praphanphoj V, Stingl JC, Tsai SJ, Kubo M, Klein TE, Weinshilboum R (2015) The International SSRI Pharmacogenomics Consortium (ISPC): a genome-wide association study of antidepressant treatment response. Transl Psychiatry 5:e553

Breen G, Li Q, Roth BL, O'Donnell P, Didriksen M, Dolmetsch R, O'Reilly PF, Gaspar HA, Manji H, Huebel C, Kelsoe JR, Malhotra D, Bertolino A, Posthuma D, Sklar P, Kapur S, Sullivan PF, Collier DA, Edenberg HJ (2016) Translating genome-wide association findings into new therapeutics for psychiatry. Nat Neurosci 19:1392–1396

Carvalho AF, Berk M, Hyphantis TN, Mcintyre RS (2014) The integrative management of treatment-resistant depression: a comprehensive review and perspectives. Psychother Psychosom 83:70–88

Caudill MM, Hunter AM, Cook IA, Leuchter AF (2015) The antidepressant treatment response index as a predictor of Reboxetine treatment outcome in major depressive disorder. Clin EEG Neurosci 46:277–284

Chekroud AM, Zotti RJ, Shehzad Z, Gueorguieva R, Johnson MK, Trivedi MH, Cannon TD, Krystal JH, Corlett PR (2016) Cross-trial prediction of treatment outcome in depression: a machine learning approach. Lancet Psychiatry 3:243–250

Chekroud AM, Gueorguieva R, Krumholz HM, Trivedi MH, Krystal JH, Mccarthy G (2017) Reevaluating the efficacy and predictability of antidepressant treatments: a symptom clustering approach. JAMA Psychiat 74:370–378

Chen CC, Schwender H, Keith J, Nunkesser R, Mengersen K, Macrossan P (2011) Methods for identifying SNP interactions: a review on variations of Logic Regression, Random Forest and Bayesian logistic regression. IEEE/ACM Trans Comput Biol Bioinform 8:1580–1591

Cipriani A, Furukawa TA, Salanti G, Chaimani A, Atkinson LZ, Ogawa Y, Leucht S, Ruhe HG, Turner EH, Higgins JPT, Egger M, Takeshima N, Hayasaka Y, Imai H, Shinohara K, Tajika A, Ioannidis JPA, Geddes JR (2018) Comparative efficacy and acceptability of 21 antidepressant drugs for the acute treatment of adults with major depressive disorder: a systematic review and network meta-analysis. Lancet 391:1357–1366

Cohen ZD, Derubeis RJ (2018) Treatment selection in depression. Annu Rev Clin Psychol 14:209–236

Costafreda SG, Chu C, Ashburner J, Fu CH (2009) Prognostic and diagnostic potential of the structural neuroanatomy of depression. PLoS One 4:e6353

Derubeis RJ, Cohen ZD, Forand NR, Fournier JC, Gelfand LA, Lorenzo-Luaces L (2014) The personalized advantage index: translating research on prediction into individualized treatment recommendations. A demonstration. PLoS One 9:e83875

Dold M, Kasper S (2016) Evidence-based pharmacotherapy of treatment-resistant unipolar depression. Int J Psychiatry Clin Pract 21:1–11

Fried EI (2017) The 52 symptoms of major depression: lack of content overlap among seven common depression scales. J Affect Disord 208:191–197

Fried EI, Van Borkulo CD, Epskamp S, Schoevers RA, Tuerlinckx F, Borsboom D (2016) Measuring depression over time. Or not? Lack of unidimensionality and longitudinal measurement invariance in four common rating scales of depression. Psychol Assess 28:1354–1367

Garcia-Gonzalez J, Tansey KE, Hauser J, Henigsberg N, Maier W, Mors O, Placentino A, Rietschel M, Souery D, Zagar T, Czerski PM, Jerman B, Buttenschon HN, Schulze TG, Zobel A, Farmer A, Aitchison KJ, Craig I, Mcguffin P, Giupponi M, Perroud N, Bondolfi G, Evans D, O'Donovan M, Peters TJ, Wendland JR, Lewis G, Kapur S, Perlis R, Arolt V, Domschke K, Breen G, Curtis C, Sang-Hyuk L, Kan C, Newhouse S, Patel H, Baune BT, Uher R, Lewis CM, Fabbri C, Major Depressive Disorder Working Group of the Psychiatric Genomic Consortium (2017) Pharmacogenetics of antidepressant response: a polygenic approach. Prog Neuropsychopharmacol Biol Psychiatry 75:128–134

Gratten J, Wray NR, Keller MC, Visscher PM (2014) Large-scale genomics unveils the genetic architecture of psychiatric disorders. Nat Neurosci 17:782–790

Grisanzio KA, Goldstein-Piekarski AN, Wang MY, Rashed Ahmed AP, Samara Z, Williams LM (2018) Transdiagnostic symptom clusters and associations with brain, behavior, and daily function in mood, anxiety, and trauma disorders. JAMA Psychiat 75:201–209

Hunter AM, Cook IA, Greenwald SD, Tran ML, Miyamoto KN, Leuchter AF (2011) The antidepressant treatment response index and treatment outcomes in a placebo-controlled trial of fluoxetine. J Clin Neurophysiol 28:478–482

Iniesta R, Malki K, Maier W, Rietschel M, Mors O, Hauser J, Henigsberg N, Dernovsek MZ, Souery D, Stahl D, Dobson R, Aitchison KJ, Farmer A, Lewis CM, Mcguffin P, Uher R (2016) Combining clinical variables to optimize prediction of antidepressant treatment outcomes. J Psychiatr Res 78:94–102

Iniesta R, Hodgson K, Stahl D, Malki K, Maier W, Rietschel M, Mors O, Hauser J, Henigsberg N, Dernovsek MZ, Souery D, Dobson R, Aitchison KJ, Farmer A, Mcguffin P, Lewis CM, Uher R (2018) Antidepressant drug-specific prediction of depression treatment outcomes from genetic and clinical variables. Sci Rep 8:5530

Jung J, Tawa EA, Muench C, Rosen AD, Rickels K, Lohoff FW (2017) Genome-wide association study of treatment response to venlafaxine XR in generalized anxiety disorder. Psychiatry Res 254:8–11

Kautzky A, Baldinger P, Souery D, Montgomery S, Mendlewicz J, Zohar J, Serretti A, Lanzenberger R, Kasper S (2015) The combined effect of genetic polymorphisms and clinical parameters on treatment outcome in treatment-resistant depression. Eur Neuropsychopharmacol 25:441–453

Kautzky A, Baldinger-Melich P, Kranz GS, Vanicek T, Souery D, Montgomery S, Mendlewicz J, Zohar J, Serretti A, Lanzenberger R, Kasper S (2017a) A new prediction model for evaluating treatment-resistant depression. J Clin Psychiatry 78:215–222

Kautzky A, Dold M, Bartova L, Spies M, Vanicek T, Souery D, Montgomery S, Mendlewicz J, Zohar J, Fabbri C, Serretti A, Lanzenberger R, Kasper S (2017b) Refining prediction in treatment-resistant depression: results of machine learning analyses in the TRD III sample. J Clin Psychiatry 79. https://doi.org/10.4088/JCP.16m11385

Kennedy SH, Downar J, Evans KR, Feilotter H, Lam RW, Macqueen GM, Milev R, Parikh SV, Rotzinger S, Soares C (2012) The Canadian biomarker integration network in depression (CAN-BIND): advances in response prediction. Curr Pharm Des 18:5976–5989

Liu F, Guo W, Yu D, Gao Q, Gao K, Xue Z, Du H, Zhang J, Tan C, Liu Z, Zhao J, Chen H (2012) Classification of different therapeutic responses of major depressive disorder with multivariate pattern analysis method based on structural MR scans. PLoS One 7:e40968

Maciukiewicz M, Marshe VS, Tiwari AK, Fonseka TM, Freeman N, Kennedy JL, Rotzinger S, Foster JA, Kennedy SH, Muller DJ (2017) Genome-wide association studies of placebo and duloxetine response in major depressive disorder. Pharmacogenomics J 18(3):406–412

Maciukiewicz M, Marshe VS, Hauschild AC, Foster JA, Rotzinger S, Kennedy JL, Kennedy SH, Muller DJ, Geraci J (2018) GWAS-based machine learning approach to predict duloxetine response in major depressive disorder. J Psychiatr Res 99:62–68

Mandelli L, Serretti A, Souery D, Mendlewicz J, Kasper S, Montgomery S, Zohar J (2016) High occupational level is associated with poor response to treatment of depression. Eur Neuropsychopharmacol 26:1320–1326

Marquand AF, Mourao-Miranda J, Brammer MJ, Cleare AJ, Fu CH (2008) Neuroanatomy of verbal working memory as a diagnostic biomarker for depression. Neuroreport 19:1507–1511

Musil R, Seemuller F, Meyer S, Spellmann I, Adli M, Bauer M, Kronmuller KT, Brieger P, Laux G, Bender W, Heuser I, Fisher R, Gaebel W, Schennach R, Moller HJ, Riedel M (2018) Subtypes of depression and their overlap in a naturalistic inpatient sample of major depressive disorder. Int J Methods Psychiatr Res 27. https://doi.org/10.1002/mpr.1569

Nouretdinov I, Costafreda SG, Gammerman A, Chervonenkis A, Vovk V, Vapnik V, Fu CH (2011) Machine learning classification with confidence: application of transductive conformal predictors to MRI-based diagnostic and prognostic markers in depression. NeuroImage 56:809–813

Passos IC, Mwangi B, Kapczinski F (2016) Big data analytics and machine learning: 2015 and beyond. Lancet Psychiatry 3:13–15

Patel MJ, Andreescu C, Price JC, Edelman KL, Reynolds CF 3rd, Aizenstein HJ (2015) Machine learning approaches for integrating clinical and imaging features in late-life depression classification and response prediction. Int J Geriatr Psychiatry 30:1056–1067

Perlis RH (2013) A clinical risk stratification tool for predicting treatment resistance in major depressive disorder. Biol Psychiatry 74:7–14

Perlis RH (2016) Abandoning personalization to get to precision in the pharmacotherapy of depression. World Psychiatry 15:228–235

Perlis RH, Fijal B, Adams DH, Sutton VK, Trivedi MH, Houston JP (2009) Variation in catechol-O-methyltransferase is associated with duloxetine response in a clinical trial for major depressive disorder. Biol Psychiatry 65:785–791

Perlis RH, Fijal B, Dharia S, Heinloth AN, Houston JP (2010) Failure to replicate genetic associations with antidepressant treatment response in duloxetine-treated patients. Biol Psychiatry 67:1110–1113

Riedel M, Moller HJ, Obermeier M, Adli M, Bauer M, Kronmuller K, Brieger P, Laux G, Bender W, Heuser I, Zeiler J, Gaebel W, Schennach-Wolff R, Henkel V, Seemuller F (2011) Clinical predictors of response and remission in inpatients with depressive syndromes. J Affect Disord 133:137–149

Scarr E, Millan MJ, Bahn S, Bertolino A, Turck CW, Kapur S, Moller HJ, Dean B (2015) Biomarkers for psychiatry: the journey from fantasy to fact, a report of the 2013 CINP think tank. Int J Neuropsychopharmacol 18:pyv042

Schmaal L, Marquand AF, Rhebergen D, Van Tol MJ, Ruhe HG, Van Der Wee NJ, Veltman DJ, Penninx BW (2015) Predicting the naturalistic course of major depressive disorder using clinical and multimodal neuroimaging information: a multivariate pattern recognition study. Biol Psychiatry 78:278–286

Schosser A, Serretti A, Souery D, Mendlewicz J, Zohar J, Montgomery S, Kasper S (2012) European Group for the Study of Resistant Depression (GSRD)—where have we gone so far: review of clinical and genetic findings. Eur Neuropsychopharmacol 22:453–468

Serretti A, Olgiati P, Liebman MN, Hu H, Zhang Y, Zanardi R, Colombo C, Smeraldi E (2007) Clinical prediction of antidepressant response in mood disorders: linear multivariate vs. neural network models. Psychiatry Res 152:223–231

Shafer AB (2006) Meta-analysis of the factor structures of four depression questionnaires: Beck, CES-D, Hamilton, and Zung. J Clin Psychol 62:123–146

Sinyor M, Schaffer A, Levitt A (2010) The sequenced treatment alternatives to relieve depression (STAR*D) trial: a review. Can J Psychiatr 55:126–135

Souery D, Oswald P, Massat I, Bailer U, Bollen J, Demyttenaere K, Kasper S, Lecrubier Y, Montgomery S, Serretti A, Zohar J, Mendlewicz J, Group for the Study of Resistant Depression (2007) Clinical factors associated with treatment resistance in major depressive disorder: results from a European multicenter study. J Clin Psychiatry 68:1062–1070

Sullivan PF, Neale MC, Kendler KS (2000) Genetic epidemiology of major depression: review and meta-analysis. Am J Psychiatry 157:1552–1562

Tansey KE, Guipponi M, Perroud N, Bondolfi G, Domenici E, Evans D, Hall SK, Hauser J, Henigsberg N, Hu X, Jerman B, Maier W, Mors O, O'Donovan M, Peters TJ, Placentino A, Rietschel M, Souery D, Aitchison KJ, Craig I, Farmer A, Wendland JR, Malafosse A, Holmans P, Lewis G, Lewis CM, Stensbol TB, Kapur S, Mcguffin P, Uher R (2012) Genetic predictors of response to serotonergic and noradrenergic antidepressants in major depressive disorder: a genome-wide analysis of individual-level data and a meta-analysis. PLoS Med 9:e1001326

Tansey KE, Guipponi M, Hu X, Domenici E, Lewis G, Malafosse A, Wendland JR, Lewis CM, Mcguffin P, Uher R (2013) Contribution of common genetic variants to antidepressant response. Biol Psychiatry 73:679–682

Ten Have M, Lamers F, Wardenaar K, Beekman A, De Jonge P, Van Dorsselaer S, Tuithof M, Kleinjan M, De Graaf R (2016) The identification of symptom-based subtypes of depression: a nationally representative cohort study. J Affect Disord 190:395–406

Thase ME (2008) Management of patients with treatment-resistant depression. J Clin Psychiatry 69:e8

Uher R, Perroud N, Ng MY, Hauser J, Henigsberg N, Maier W, Mors O, Placentino A, Rietschel M, Souery D, Zagar T, Czerski PM, Jerman B, Larsen ER, Schulze TG, Zobel A, Cohen-Woods S, Pirlo K, Butler AW, Muglia P, Barnes MR, Lathrop M, Farmer A, Breen G, Aitchison KJ, Craig I, Lewis CM, Mcguffin P (2010) Genome-wide pharmacogenetics of antidepressant response in the GENDEP project. Am J Psychiatry 167:555–564

Ulbricht CM, Rothschild AJ, Lapane KL (2015) The association between latent depression subtypes and remission after treatment with citalopram: a latent class analysis with distal outcome. J Affect Disord 188:270–277

Ulbricht CM, Dumenci L, Rothschild AJ, Lapane KL (2016) Changes in depression subtypes for women during treatment with citalopram: a latent transition analysis. Arch Womens Ment Health 19:769–778

Ulbricht CM, Dumenci L, Rothschild AJ, Lapane KL (2018) Changes in depression subtypes among men in STAR*D: a latent transition analysis. Am J Mens Health 12:5–13

Van Loo HM, De Jonge P, Romeijn JW, Kessler RC, Schoevers RA (2012) Data-driven subtypes of major depressive disorder: a systematic review. BMC Med 10:156

Van Loo HM, Cai T, Gruber MJ, Li J, De Jonge P, Petukhova M, Rose S, Sampson NA, Schoevers RA, Wardenaar KJ, Wilcox MA, Al-Hamzawi AO, Andrade LH, Bromet EJ, Bunting B, Fayyad J, Florescu SE, Gureje O, Hu C, Huang Y, Levinson D, Medina-Mora ME, Nakane Y, Posada-Villa J, Scott KM, Xavier M, Zarkov Z, Kessler RC (2014) Major depressive disorder subtypes to predict long-term course. Depress Anxiety 31:765–777

Vassos E, Di Forti M, Coleman J, Iyegbe C, Prata D, Euesden J, O'Reilly P, Curtis C, Kolliakou A, Patel H, Newhouse S, Traylor M, Ajnakina O, Mondelli V, Marques TR, Gardner-Sood P, Aitchison KJ, Powell J, Atakan Z, Greenwood KE, Smith S, Ismail K, Pariante C, Gaughran F, Dazzan P, Markus HS, David AS, Lewis CM, Murray RM, Breen G (2017) An examination of polygenic score risk prediction in individuals with first-episode psychosis. Biol Psychiatry 81:470–477

Wanders RB, Van Loo HM, Vermunt JK, Meijer RR, Hartman CA, Schoevers RA, Wardenaar KJ, De Jonge P (2016) Casting wider nets for anxiety and depression: disability-driven cross-diagnostic subtypes in a large cohort. Psychol Med 46:3371–3382

Wardenaar KJ, Van Loo HM, Cai T, Fava M, Gruber MJ, Li J, De Jonge P, Nierenberg AA, Petukhova MV, Rose S, Sampson NA, Schoevers RA, Wilcox MA, Alonso J, Bromet EJ, Bunting B, Florescu SE, Fukao A, Gureje O, Hu C, Huang YQ, Karam AN, Levinson D, Medina Mora ME, Posada-Villa J, Scott KM, Taib NI, Viana MC, Xavier M, Zarkov Z, Kessler RC (2014) The effects of co-morbidity in defining major depression subtypes associated with long-term course and severity. Psychol Med 44:3289–3302

WHO (2001) World health report 2001. Mental health—new understanding, new hope. WHO, Geneva

The Role of Big Data Analytics in Predicting Suicide

5

Ronald C. Kessler, Samantha L. Bernecker, Robert M. Bossarte, Alex R. Luedtke, John F. McCarthy, Matthew K. Nock, Wilfred R. Pigeon, Maria V. Petukhova, Ekaterina Sadikova, Tyler J. VanderWeele, Kelly L. Zuromski, and Alan M. Zaslavsky

This chapter reviews the long history of using electronic medical records and other types of big data to predict suicide. Although a number of the most recent of these studies used machine learning (ML) methods, these studies were all suboptimal both in the features used as predictors and in the analytic approaches used to develop the prediction models. We review these limitations and describe opportunities for making improvements in future applications. We also review the controversy among clinical experts about using structured suicide risk assessment tools (be they based on ML or older prediction methods) versus in-depth clinical evaluations of needs for treatment planning. Rather than seeing them as competitors, we propose integrating

R. C. Kessler (✉) · M. V. Petukhova · E. Sadikova · A. M. Zaslavsky
Department of Health Care Policy, Harvard Medical School, Boston, MA, USA
e-mail: Kessler@hcp.med.harvard.edu

S. L. Bernecker · M. K. Nock · K. L. Zuromski
Department of Psychology, Harvard University, Cambridge, MA, USA

R. M. Bossarte · W. R. Pigeon
Departments of Behavioral Medicine and Psychiatry, West Virginia University School of Medicine, Morgantown, WV, USA

U.S. Department of Veterans Affairs Center of Excellence for Suicide Prevention, Canandaigua, NY, USA

A. R. Luedtke
Vaccine and Infectious Disease Division, Fred Hutchinson Cancer Research Center, Seattle, WA, USA

J. F. McCarthy
Serious Mental Illness Treatment Resource and Evaluation Center, Office of Mental Health Operations, VA Center for Clinical Management Research, Ann Arbor, MI, USA

T. J. VanderWeele
Department of Biostatistics, Harvard T.H. Chan School of Public Health, Boston, MA, USA

Department of Epidemiology, Harvard T.H. Chan School of Public Health, Boston, MA, USA

I. C. Passos et al., *Personalized Psychiatry*,
https://doi.org/10.1007/978-3-030-03553-2_5

these different approaches to capitalize on their complementary strengths. We also emphasize the distinction between two types of ML analyses: those aimed at predicting which patients are at highest suicide risk, and those aimed at predicting the treatment options that will be best for individual patients. We explain why both are needed to optimize the value of big data ML methods in addressing the suicide problem.

5.1 Introduction

Suicide is the 17th leading cause of death in the world (approximately 800,000 suicides per year) and the second leading cause of death among 15–29 year olds (World Health Organization [WHO] 2018a). The actual number of suicides is likely to be higher, as some suicides are misclassified as accidental deaths (Katz et al. 2016). Psychological autopsy studies find that up to 90% of people who died by suicide in Western countries met criteria for a mental disorder (Joiner et al. 2017). In addition, up to 90% of suicide decedents in Western countries came into contact with the healthcare system in the year before death, up to two-thirds had a mental health treatment contact during that year, up to 30% had a psychiatric hospitalization or emergency department visit for a psychiatric problem during that year, and up to one-third were in mental health treatment in the month before death (Ahmedani et al. 2014; Luoma et al. 2002; Pearson et al. 2009; Schaffer et al. 2016). This high level of contact with the healthcare system represents a major opportunity to improve detection of suicide risk in health care settings and target interventions that substantially reduce suicides (Berman and Silverman 2014).

The value of systematically quantifying suicide risk has been debated for over 60 years. In 1954, Rosen argued that the low incidence of suicide poses a substantial barrier, "for in the attempt to predict suicide or any other infrequent event, a large number of false positives are obtained," which means that "such an index would have no practical value, for it would be impossible to treat as potential suicides the prodigious number of false positives" and treating only those at highest risk as potential suicides would miss the majority of true positives. Murphy (1972) countered that the practicality of suicide risk prediction depends on "what is considered appropriate treatment for persons at increased risk of suicide." This debate has continued since these early commentaries at the same time that empirical research has been carried out to improve prediction models and address the problems of false positives and false negatives. Recent studies have used machine learning (ML) methods to develop these models. We begin our review of the literature with a consideration of earlier studies on risk factors for suicide among hospital inpatients and other high-risk patients. We then discuss the ongoing controversy about using structured suicide risk assessment tools. We then review recent studies that used ML methods to predict suicide risk. Finally, we close with recommendations for future studies.

5.2 Earlier Multivariate Analyses Predicting Suicide Among Inpatients

Due to the rarity and short duration of most psychiatric hospitalizations, the proportion of all suicides that occurs among psychiatric inpatients is estimated to be no more than about 5% (Madsen et al. 2017). However, conditional suicide risk among psychiatric inpatients is nonetheless high, especially during the times they are out on temporary leave, with a recent meta-analysis estimating this rate to be 147/100,000 inpatient-years (Walsh et al. 2015) compared to a global population-wide age-standardized suicide rate of 10.7/100,000 person-years (WHO 2018b). Another recent meta-analysis reviewed the 17 studies published between 1998 and 2016 that carried out multivariate analyses of clinical risk factors to predict inpatient suicides (Large et al. 2017a). These studies all used either a cohort design or a retrospective case-control design and focused on predictors extracted from medical records, although one research group also obtained data from a retrospective questionnaire sent to treating psychiatrists. A total of 191,944 inpatients were included in these pooled studies, 1718 (0.9%) of whom died by suicide while hospitalized. The mean number of predictors considered in the studies was 78.6 (14–272 range) and the mean number in the final models was 6.1.

The methods used in developing these models likely resulted in over-fitting, as in the majority of cases univariate logistic regression analysis was used to select a subset of predictors for subsequent multivariate logistic analysis and a liberal *p* value was often used in selecting predictors for multivariate analysis. The multivariate analysis typically used backward stepwise selection to arrive at a parsimonious final model. No cross-validation was used to adjust for over-fitting. Recursive partitioning was used in a few studies to search for interactions, but again with no cross-validation, and the analyses otherwise assumed additivity. The focus of all the studies was on identifying "high-risk" patients by defining a threshold, typically on the individual-level predicted probability scale based on the final model, although in some cases the threshold was based on a count of dichotomously-scored predictors with positive values. We were unable to discover a principled basis for selecting thresholds in any of these studies even after a careful review of the original reports, such as to maximize sensitivity (SN; the proportion of suicides that occurred among patients classified as being above the risk threshold) for a fixed specificity (SP; the proportion of patients not dying by suicide that were classified correctly as being below the risk threshold), to equalize SN and SP, to equalize the number of false positives and the number of false negatives, or to equalize the number of false positives and r times the number of false negatives (where $r =$ the pre-specified relative importance of false positives versus false negatives).

Although the great variety of predictors and thresholds used in these studies makes it impossible to draw firm conclusions about prediction accuracy, the authors of the meta-analysis used a random-effects model to generate a meta-analytic ROC curve across studies. SN was estimated to be about 0.70 when SP was set at 0.80 and about 0.50 when SP was set at 0.90. Given the relatively short duration of most hospitalizations, positive predictive value (PPV; the incidence of suicide among patients classified as high-risk) was only about 0.004, but this was roughly 10 times as high as the suicide rate among patients classified below the threshold. The authors of the meta-analysis concluded from these results that risk assessment based on multivariate prediction models "is not useful as a basis of clinical decisions." Two observations were made to support this conclusion: first, that the low PPV meant that special interventions for high-risk patients would "subject many patients, who will never suicide, to excessive intrusion or coercion"; and second, that the low SN meant that patients classified as being low-risk account for a substantial proportion of inpatient suicides.

This rejection of standardized suicide risk prediction tools is consistent with the recommendations made in a number of other recent systematic reviews, meta-analyses, and commentaries (Bolton 2015; Bolton et al. 2015; Carter et al. 2017; Chan et al. 2016; Katz et al. 2017; Larkin et al. 2014; Mulder et al. 2016; Owens and Kelley 2017; Quinlivan et al. 2016; Runeson et al. 2017). This might seem to be inconsistent with clinical practice guidelines that call for mental health professionals always to make suicide risk evaluations of psychiatric inpatients and patients presenting with psychiatric crises in emergency departments (Bernert et al. 2014; Silverman et al. 2015). However, these guidelines typically advise against using structured risk prediction tools for this purpose and instead recommend that clinicians "initiate a therapeutic relationship" to make "an integrated and comprehensive psychosocial assessment" of needs and risks (National Institute for Health and Care Excellence [NICE] 2011; O'Connor et al. 2013). The notion here is that the low SN of structured suicide risk tools requires clinicians to consider all inpatients and patients in psychiatric crisis to be at risk of suicide and to focus on treatment needs rather than attempt to distinguish levels of risk.

5.3 Earlier Multivariate Analyses Predicting Suicide Among Other High-Risk Patients

Other empirical studies have been carried out for many years to predict suicide and attempted suicide in two other partly-overlapping high-risk patient populations: psychiatric inpatients after hospital discharge, and patients presenting to emergency departments after nonfatal suicide attempts (whether or not they were subsequently hospitalized). The pooled suicide rate within the first 3 months after psychiatric hospital discharge was estimated in a recent meta-analysis of these studies to be 1132/100,000 person-years, with successively lower cumulative rates in studies that followed patients 3–12 months (654/100,000 person-years), 1–5 years (494/100,000 person-years), 6–10 years (366/100,000 person-years), and more than 10 years (277/100,000 person-years) (Chung et al. 2017), although none of the individual studies that followed patients over long time periods estimated changes in conditional risk over shorter time periods. Another recent meta-analysis that focused on suicide after self-harm (whether or not the patient was hospitalized) estimated a pooled suicide incidence within 1 year of the index self-harm episode of 1600/100,000, with higher estimates of cumulative incidence in studies that followed patients 2 years (2100/100,000), 5 years (3900/100,000), and 10 years (4200/100,000) (Carroll et al. 2014).

As detailed in several recent systematic reviews and meta-analyses (Bolton et al. 2015; Carter et al. 2017; Chan et al. 2016; Katz et al. 2017; Larkin et al. 2014; Quinlivan et al. 2016; Runeson et al. 2017), these studies were usually based on designs similar to the studies reviewed above on inpatient suicides: that is, either cohort or retrospective case-control designs, with predictors extracted from clinical records, although some studies also used patient self-report scales as predictors. The follow-up periods varied widely (6 months to 5 years). Some studies used survival analysis to study predictors over variable time periods, but no systematic effort was made in these studies to investigate change in relative importance of predictors by length of follow-up. The absence of the latter focus is a weakness because suicide risk is known to be highest shortly after clinical contact and there have been calls for increased focus on prediction during high-risk periods (Glenn and Nock 2014; Olfson et al. 2014). It was rare for risk factor analyses in these or other studies to focus on the relatively short 30-day risk window of most interest to clinicians (Franklin et al. 2017).

Some studies evaluating suicide risk prediction tools in high-risk populations were based on single scales, such as self-report scales of hopelessness (Beck and Steer 1988), depression (Beck et al. 1996), overall psychopathological severity (Lindqvist et al. 2007), suicide intent (Beck et al. 1974), and attitudes toward suicide (Koldsland et al. 2012). Other studies used multivariate prediction equations to develop composite suicide risk tools. The latter studies typically began with a predictor set, often extracted from clinical records and sometimes also including various patient self-report and clinician rating scales, used preliminary univariate analyses to select a reduced subset of significant predictors, and then formed a composite from these predictors. Trial and error cross-tabulations (e.g., Kreitman and Foster 1991) and considerations of content validity (e.g., Patterson et al. 1983) were used to construct most of the earlier tools of this sort. Logistic regression analysis or survival analysis were used to construct most of the more recently-developed empirically-derived suicide prediction tools. The predictors in some of these tools consisted entirely of socio-demographic and clinical data extracted from electronic medical records (e.g., Spittal et al. 2014), but others also included some of the patient-reported scales described above (e.g., Bilen et al. 2013; Randall et al. 2013). A few recently-developed empirically-derived tools were constructed using recursive partitioning (Cooper et al. 2006; Steeg et al. 2012; Steinberg and Phillip 1997). As in the inpatient suicide studies, single high-risk thresholds were typically specified without clear evidence of a principled basis for threshold selection, resulting in a wide range in the proportion of patients classified as being high risk. Even though the tools developed in these studies often significantly predicted subsequent suicide, reviews and meta-analyses consistently concluded, as in the inpatient studies, that operating characteristics (i.e., SN, SP, PPV) were not sufficiently strong to justify using any of these tools as a basis for clinical decision-making.

5.4 Reconsidering the Rationale for Rejecting Standardized Suicide Prediction Tools

As noted above, critics of standardized suicide risk prediction tools emphasize the fact that these tools have relatively low PPV and SN, leading clinicians to draw "false reassurance" when they use these tools in treatment planning, patients incorrectly classified as high-risk to experience needless intrusion or coercion, and patients incorrectly classified as low-risk to be denied the treatment they need. Critics also argue that patients perceive standardized risk prediction tools as superficial and that this perception interferes with establishing the kind of therapeutic alliance needed to carry out a more in-depth clinical risk assessment (Large et al. 2017b; Mulder et al. 2016; Owens and Kelley 2017). Qualitative studies debriefing UK patients who were administered standardized scales are said to be consistent with the latter concern (Hunter et al. 2013; Owens et al. 2016; Palmer et al. 2007; Taylor et al. 2009).

Arguments can be made against each of these criticisms. With regard to low PPV: Even though it is true that patients incorrectly classified as high-risk would experience additional burden by being treated if they were at high risk, a balance needs to be struck between increased intrusion-coercion for, say, 250 patients (1/0.004; the number of false positives for every true positive when PPV = 0.004, as in the Large et al. meta-analysis cited above) incorrectly classified as high-risk and saving one life. It is not at all obvious that a formal cost-benefit analysis would conclude that the cost-benefit ratio is >1.0 in such a case. In addition, recent studies have found that up to one-third of patients who do not die by suicide but are classified as high-risk are also at high risk of other experiences in the same spectrum, such as deaths classified as accidental or undetermined, nonfatal suicide attempts, serious nonfatal injuries classified as accidental, and psychiatric hospitalizations (Kessler et al. 2015; McCarthy et al. 2015). The potential to reduce incidence of these outcomes would increase the cost-effectiveness of interventions.

With regard to low SN: The suicide risk models reviewed above all searched for high-risk thresholds (i.e., thresholds to maximize SN for a given SP). There is no way to know from such analyses if a useful threshold could be specified for low-risk patients (i.e., a threshold to maximize SP for SN close to 1.0). Reanalysis, which would have to use the original data in each study, might find that a substantial proportion of patients could be isolated that had such a vanishingly small suicide risk that they could be spared the burden of further evaluation. Indeed, as elaborated below, we believe that this search for a practical low-risk threshold should be the main focus of a first-stage in a multi-stage ML analysis of suicide risk.

With regard to the claim that patients perceive structured suicide risk assessments as superficial: This claim implies that use of clinical suicide risk evaluations instead of standardized suicide risk prediction tools leads to increased detection of suicidality. However, we are aware of no experimental evaluation of this hypothesis. We do know, though, that one study found that clinicians asked to predict the likelihood that patients they are evaluating for suicide risk in at Emergency Departments (ED) will make a suicide attempt over the next 6 months were no better than chance in their predictions (Nock et al. 2010). This suggests that detailed clinical evaluations might not be as helpful in this regard as implied by critics of standardized risk assessments. A recent systematic review is broadly consistent with this view in finding that clinical risk evaluations are not strong predictors of subsequent suicidal behaviors (Woodford et al. 2017).

In addition, there is evidence that in some cases a structured suicide risk assessment yields better predictions than a clinical evaluation. In an early study on the use of computerized screening for suicide risk, patients in a crisis intervention clinic were asked to complete a computerized assessment of suicidality and then asked whether they would have preferred to have given this information directly to a doctor or to the computer (Greist et al. 1973). The majority of patients said they preferred to provide the information to the computer. A subsequent study building on this finding used a series of computerized self-report questions to assess hospitalized patients who had been admitted because of suicide attempts and then had a psychiatrist carry out an independent face-to-face evaluation blinded to patient reports on the computerized assessment (Levine et al. 1989). Retrospective comparisons showed that patients who subsequently engaged in suicidal behaviors were more likely to admit sensitive symptoms to the computer than to the psychiatrist. This finding is consistent with a good deal of experimental research showing that the likelihood of reporting embarrassing or stigmatizing thoughts and behaviors increases when respondents are randomized to more confidential modes of reporting (Brown et al. 2013; Gnambs and Kaspar 2015). Based on the above results, a computerized version of the self-report Columbia Suicide Severity Rating Scale (CSSRS; Posner et al. 2011) was developed and administered to 6760 patients with psychiatric disorders and 2077 patients with physical disorders who participated in 33 different prospective clinical research studies (Greist et al. 2014). The vast majority (89.9%) of subsequent suicidal behaviors were predicted accurately by the CSSRS.

These results are important given that detailed clinical suicide risk evaluations are carried out only with slightly more than half of all psychiatric inpatients and ED patients in psychiatric crises even when official policies call for these evaluations to be carried out (Cooper et al. 2013). Furthermore, structured suicide risk assessment tools continue to be widely used even when clinical practice guidelines explicitly suggest that they not be used (Quinlivan et al. 2014). Why? One possibility is that the time-consuming nature of detailed clinical suicide risk evaluations leads them to be used only selectively. Gold-standard clinical evaluations of this sort are very time-consuming, often requiring multiple sessions (Rudd 2014) to assess needs (e.g., mental and physical health problems, life difficulties, reasons for recent self-harm and for possible future self-harm, and needs for diverse interventions) and risks (e.g., the nature of the patient's suicidal thinking and behaviors, predispositions to suicide, previous suicide attempts, hopelessness, impulsivity/self-control, suicide warning signs for imminent risk, and protective factors).

How is the decision made to carry out these detailed evaluations with some patients but not others? We are aware of no discussion of this question in the literature. One possibility worth considering is that standardized suicide prediction tools might be useful in helping clinicians make this decision. Not enough research has been focused on this possibility to know how helpful existing tools could be in this respect, but, as noted below, the small amount of existing evidence suggests that this might be a fruitful direction for future research. The goal would be to define a *low-risk* (not high-risk) threshold for patients who would not be subjected to a more in-depth clinical risk evaluation because of the low proportion of actual suicides that occurs among such patients. If a ML-based decision support tool based on a structured assessment battery could be developed of this sort, one that yielded a meaningful SP for a SN near 1.0, it would almost certainly improve substantially on whatever current decision rules clinicians are using in deciding which patients to evaluate and which not.

It is clear from the results of recent prospective studies that any such assessment battery would have to go beyond patient self-reports of suicidality. These studies have shown that a substantial proportion of the patients who went on to die by suicide shortly after making healthcare visits denied being suicidal during those visits when asked explicitly about suicidality (Louzon et al. 2016; Simon et al. 2013). However, a number of novel structured self-report suicide risk assessment tools developed recently have been shown to have higher predictive validity than previously-developed tools and to be predictive among patients who deny being suicidal. These new tools include: performance-based neurocognitive tests of suicide-related implicit cognitions (Nock et al. 2010); self-reports of suicide-related beliefs (Bryan et al. 2014) and volitional factors such as fearlessness of death, impulsivity, and exposure to past suicidal behaviors (Dhingra et al. 2015); and tools based on linguistic and acoustic features extracted from tape-recorded responses to open-ended questions that do not ask about suicidality (Pestian et al. 2017). It is also worthwhile remembering that previously-developed structured suicide prediction tools measure many of the same dimensions that guidelines call for including in detailed clinical suicide risk evaluations and that these structured tools have been shown to be significant predictors of subsequent suicidal behaviors even though they are not sufficiently strong predictors when considered one at a time to guide clinical decision-making (Bolton et al. 2015; Carter et al. 2017). It is plausible to think that a comprehensive computerized battery that includes all these measures along with the detailed EMR data used in the recent ML prediction models reviewed below would be able to define a low-risk segment of the patient population that had a sufficiently low predicted risk of suicide not to receive a subsequent in-depth clinical evaluation.

Although we are aware of no attempt to develop a comprehensive structured predictor battery of this sort, encouraging results have been found in studies that administered a small number of structured suicide risk tools and found that prediction accuracy is improved significantly by combining them rather than considering them one at a time (Randall et al. 2013; Stefansson et al. 2015). It would not be difficult to expand this line of investigation with existing data. For example, Quinlivan et al. (2017) administered seven commonly-used structured suicide risk assessment tools to a sample of patients who were referred to liaison psychiatry following suicide attempts and followed those patients for 6 months to evaluate the predictive validity of each tool for repeat suicide attempts or suicide deaths. Four of the eight tools had statistically significant odds-ratios (ORs = 3.9–8.7). Yet the researchers nonetheless concluded that "risk scales on their own have little role in the management of suicidal behavior" (Reutfors et al. 2010). This conclusion was drawn even though no attempt was made to combine the significant scales into a multivariate composite that might have had better prediction accuracy than the individual scales considered one at a time. This negative conclusion is also curious in that the same researchers noted that defining a low-risk threshold might be useful by stating that "(t)he use of risk scales is dependent on clinical context. For example, clinicians may prefer scales with high sensitivity for screening or ruling out a risk of a condition, or scales high in specificity for later stages of assessment or ruling in patients for treatment." Yet the thresholds used in their analysis were for the most part high-risk thresholds, making it impossible to draw any conclusions about the value of the tools reviewed in defining a low-risk patient subgroup.

5.5 Machine Learning Analyses Predicting Suicide Among High-Risk Patients

A number of recent studies have extended the approaches taken in the high-risk multivariate predictor studies reviewed above by using ML methods instead of logistic regression. Results show that ML methods have a great deal of promise in predicting suicide even though all the studies carried out so far have limitations that we review later in the chapter. These studies focused on suicides among psychiatric inpatients in the 12 months after hospital discharge (Kessler et al. 2015), suicides among psychiatric outpatients in the 12 months after visits (Kessler et al. 2017b), and suicide attempts in the 12 months after receiving a formal suicide risk assessment among patients in a psychiatric hospital or ED who were deemed to be at sufficiently high risk to receive such an assessment (Tran et al. 2014). The sample sizes ranged from a low of 68 post-hospitalization suicides among 53,760 hospitalized patients (Kessler et al. 2015) to a high of 1562 serious suicide attempts among 7399 patients who received suicide risk assessments (Tran et al. 2014).

All these studies used electronic medical record (EMR) data as predictors, defined a clear retrospective data capture time period for feature aggregation (2–5 years before baseline), allowed for strength of associations to vary by length of retrospective time period and time-since-baseline, used a multi-step process of feature transformation and pruning based on cross-validation in a training sample followed by evaluation in a separate validation sample, and used standard over-sampling or up-weighting of cases (He and Garcia 2009) in the training sample to deal with the problem of extreme class imbalance. Two of the studies used preliminary bootstrap recursive partitioning to search for interactions, and all the studies used some form of penalized logistic regression (either lasso or elastic net) to estimate the final model. All of the studies evaluated model performance by examining SN and PPV at predefined levels of SN and focused on high-risk prediction. One of the studies compared the prediction accuracy of the ML model with that of a structured suicide risk assessment and found that prediction based on the former was substantially better than prediction based on the latter (Tran et al. 2014).

Several of the studies suggested that their results had clinical implications. One found that more than 50% of the suicides in the year after psychiatric hospitalization among US Army personnel occurred among the 5% of inpatients classified by ML at the time of hospital discharge as being at highest suicide risk (Kessler et al. 2015). Although PPV was only 3.8%, more than one-third of these highest-risk patients experienced at least one other extreme negative outcome, such as death judged to be accidental or unclassifiable, serious nonfatal injury, attempted suicide, or repeat psychiatric hospitalization, leading the authors to suggest that it might be cost-effective to target patients defined by the ML classifier as being highest-risk for the type of intensive post-hospital case management program that is recommended but not mandated by the US Department of Defense (VA Office of Inspector General 2007). Another US Army study found that an ML model was able to isolate a small number of soldiers (about 500 out of an Army of 500,000) that accounted for a very high proportion of all suicides in the five-week high-risk period after index psychiatric outpatient visits (1047.1/100,000 person-years), leading to a recommendation to target these highest-risk outpatients to receive one of the evidence-based psychotherapies that have been developed specifically to treat suicidality (Jobes et al. 2015).

5.6 Machine Learning Analyses Predicting Suicide in Total Patient Populations

Other ML studies have attempted to predict future suicides or suicide attempts among all patients in a healthcare system (Barak-Corren et al. 2017; Ben-Ari and Hammond 2015; Choi et al. 2018; Kessler et al. 2017a; Walsh et al. 2017). Samples in these studies were typically quite large. Barak-Corren et al. (2017), for example, developed a ML model to predict future suicide attempts ($n = 20{,}246$) in a commercial health system based on an analysis of 1.7 M patients followed for up to 15 years (9.0 M person-years). Kessler et al. (2017a) developed a ML model to predict suicide deaths among patients in the US Veterans Affairs health system, the Veterans Health Administration (VHA), in 2009–2011 using a person-month data array that included information at the month before death for all 6360 VHA suicide decedents and a 1% time-matched person-month probability sample of 2,112,008 VHA service users alive at the end of an index control month over those years. This analysis built on an earlier proof-of-concept model (McCarthy et al. 2015).

As with the high-risk studies reviewed in the previous subsection, the total-population studies used structured EMR data as predictors. One also used natural language processing (NLP) methods to define features based on information extracted from clinical notes (Ben-Ari and Hammond 2015). All studies defined a clear retrospective data capture time period for feature aggregation (2–5 years), and most, but not all, cases allowed for strength of associations to vary by length of retrospective time frame and time-since-baseline. They all defined a clear risk time horizon (between 30 days and 15 years). They all used a multi-step process of feature transformation and pruning based on cross-validation in a training sample followed by testing in a separate validation sample. Most of the studies used over-sampling or up-weighting of cases in the training sample to deal with the problem of extreme class imbalance. Although analyses were consistently based on a single algorithm (artificial neural networks, naïve Bayes, penalized regression, random forests), some studies compared results across different classifiers before selecting a best one defined in terms of mean-squared error (e.g., adaptive splines, Bayesian additive regression trees, generalized boosting, support vector machines). Most, but not all, studies evaluated model performance by examining SN and PPV at predefined levels of SN, and all studies focused on high-risk assessment aimed at targeting preventive interventions rather than on low-risk assessment aimed at limiting the number of patients who would receive more in-depth clinical evaluations.

For the most part, lift (i.e., incidence of the outcome among patients classified as high-risk versus in the total patient population) was relatively high at the upper ends of the prediction scales in these studies, with SN at a fixed SP of 0.95 equal to 0.28 in the VHA suicide study (Kessler et al. 2017a) and in the range 0.28–0.50 (Barak-Corren et al. 2017; Ben-Ari and Hammond 2015) in the studies predicting suicide attempts. PPV, of course, was quite low at these thresholds due to the rarity of the outcomes. Despite the models not focusing on low-risk prediction, the 25% of patients with the lowest predicted risk in a number of these studies (Barak-Corren et al. 2017; Ben-Ari and Hammond 2015) accounted for very low (3–7%) proportions of suicidal outcomes.

5.7 Other Machine Learning Studies Aimed at Predicting Suicidality

Another group of ML studies attempted to predict either current or past patient self-reported suicidality from information obtained in administrative records and/or patient self-report scales (e.g., Barros et al. 2017; Hettige et al. 2017; Ilgen et al. 2009; Jordan et al. 2018; Oh et al. 2017; Passos et al. 2016). The rationale for these efforts was that model predictions might help unobtrusively to detect "unseen" cases of suicidality when applied in other samples. A related series of studies applied ML methods to complex feature sets made up of various biomarkers in order to predict current self-reported suicidality, using such predictors as immune markers (Dickerson et al. 2017) and altered fMRI neural signatures in response to life- and death-related words (Just et al. 2017). Other related studies used text analysis to extract predictive information from clinical notes (McCoy et al. 2016; Poulin et al. 2014) or new technologies, such as smartphones and wearable sensors that might allow passive monitoring of suicidality (Braithwaite et al. 2016; Cook et al. 2016). Samples in all these studies were small because of the high expense of the biomarkers and/or new technologies. The analyses typically used only a single ML classifier rather than an ensemble, although some studies compared results across different classifiers. Relatively simple feature selection methods were used in most of these applications. Little was said in most of them about the methods used for hyper-parameter tuning or dealing with the problem of class imbalance. Most applications used internal cross-validation but did not divide their small samples into separate training and validation sets. Practical prediction accuracy (i.e., estimates of SN or PPV for fixed high values of SN) was seldom emphasized, although overall prediction strength (AUC) was typically moderate, suggesting that these methods would be most useful if combined with administrative data to create a rich multivariate feature set.

5.8 Future Directions in Using ML for Suicide Risk Prediction

Although the studies reviewed above suggest that ML methods have considerable promise in predicting suicide, the field has as yet not fully realized that promise. A number of changes would likely improve prediction accuracy and clinical value. First, as illustrated in the last section, the feature sets used in the ML analyses of suicide carried out until now could be expanded beyond the structured EMR data that have so far been the mainstay of these analyses. In addition to the methods described in the last section, information on residential zip code could be used to extract small area geocode data from public sources on a number of important predictors of suicide such as local unemployment rates (Nordt et al. 2015) and neighborhood social capital (Holtkamp and Weaver 2018). Data from commercial search engines could be used to obtain more detailed socio-demographic information than the information on age, sex, and marital status typically available in EMRs and to extract information from public records on individual-level legal, financial, and criminal justice experiences that predict suicide (e.g., Accurint 2018).

Second, prediction accuracy could be improved by using ensemble ML methods combining individual-level predictions across algorithms. The Super Learner ensemble method, for example, has been shown to yield considerably higher levels of prediction accuracy than the best-performing algorithm in the ensemble (Polley et al. 2016). Automated machine learning (AutoML; Feurer et al. 2015; Olson et al. 2017) is also making it increasingly possible to refine feature transformation-pruning, algorithm selection, and hyperparameter tuning (Urbanowicz et al. 2017). AutoML can also be used to address the extreme imbalance problem by automatically implementing toolkits to evaluate the relative effectiveness of different imbalance correction methods (e.g., Chawla 2010).

Third, greater consideration is needed of the clinical value of different outcome time horizons in light of the fact that several studies have shown that optimal model features and coefficients differ depending on time horizon. In the ideal case, the time horizon would be chosen in light of the intervention the model is being designed to guide. This does not always occur. For example, the ML analysis described earlier predicting suicide among users of the VHA system was designed to facilitate

VHA implementation of their Recovery Engagement And Coordination for Health-Veterans Enhanced Treatment (REACH VET) program (VA Office of Public and Intergovernmental Affairs 2017) among highest-risk VHA users. However, the ML model had a 30-day time horizon even though it often takes more than 30 days to make initial contact with the targeted Veteran and the program continues for at least 90 days. This raises the question whether the REACH VET ML model should have had a longer (e.g., 180-day) time horizon and, if so, the extent to which different Veterans would have been selected for intervention if this had been done.

Fourth, ML modeling efforts need to be better coordinated with the clinical interventions they are designed to support in ways other than time horizon. Most notably, ML model development up to now has focused on high-risk prediction even though a good argument could be made that models based on the feature sets considered up to now are likely to be more useful in low-risk prediction. If that is the case, then, as suggested earlier in the chapter, a first-stage ML model based on structured predictors could be used to help select which patients should receive more intensive clinical suicide risk evaluations.

Fifth, more work needs to be done to determine the extent to which high-risk predictions based on ML models could be improved by adding information from subsequently-administered structured and/or clinical risk evaluations. Tran et al. (2014) had an opportunity to do something along these lines by virtue of the fact that their sample consisted exclusively of patients who had been the subjects of in-depth clinical suicide risk assessments, but the authors focused instead on the extent to which predictions based on ML outperformed predictions based on clinical evaluations rather than seeing how much overall prediction improved by combining the two sets of predictors.

5.9 Machine Learning Models for Clinical Decision Support in Treatment Planning

We noted above that critics of structured suicide risk prediction tools argue that all psychiatric inpatients and ED patients should be considered at risk of suicide and should receive in-depth clinical evaluations rather than structured suicide risk assessments. But this raises the question how the information about needs should be applied to formulate a treatment plan. A number of special types of psychotherapy exist for patients at high suicide risk (e.g., Jobes et al. 2017; Linehan et al. 2015; Rudd et al. 2015) that have been shown to improve on usual care in reducing suicidal behavior (Jobes et al. 2015). However, these interventions are more labor-intensive than usual care and require special clinical training, making it important to have some principled basis for knowing which patients need these interventions. The same could be said for the decision to offer combined pharmacotherapy and psychotherapy (versus only one), which is known to be of value for some but not all patients (Kessler 2018), and the use of ketamine as a pharmacologic treatment for patients at imminent suicide risk (Wilkinson and Sanacora 2016). How do clinicians make decisions about what suicidal patients need after carrying out in-depth suicide needs assessments? Critics of structured suicide risk prediction tools are silent on this question.

ML has the potential to provide clinical decision support in making these decisions, but in doing so it needs to be recognized that the patients at highest suicide risk are not necessarily the patients most likely to be helped by available interventions. This means that different ML modeling strategies need to be used to predict differential treatment response than to predict differential risk. Speaking in general terms, the models for differential treatment response can be thought of as evaluating interactions between *prescriptive* predictors of treatment response (i.e., predictors of greater response to some types of treatment than others) and treatment type, ideally evaluated in controlled treatment effectiveness trials that have real-world validity (Cohen and DeRubeis 2018). A difficulty arises, though, when the number of prescriptive predictors is large and/or when the functional forms of the interactions are complex, in which case conventional estimation methods break down. ML methods can be used in these cases (VanderWeele et al. 2018). ML methods can be applied even when treatment is not randomly assigned by using double-robust estimation methods (Vermeulen and Vansteelandt 2015), so long as either strong predictors exist of nonrandom treatment assignment or if, as in the case of suicide, loss to follow-up outcome assessment is low (Luedtke and van der Laan 2016).

To illustrate the potential value of this approach, consider the VHA's REACH VET initiative. This initiative was implemented in 2016 based on the results of an ML model that used 2008–2011 data. A separate prescriptive ML model to evaluate differential response to the REACH VET intervention could be estimated by predicting suicide deaths among high-risk VHA patients in the 12 months after selection by the initial ML intervention targeting model in 2014 (2 years before the intervention was initiated, which means that none of these high-risk patients received the intervention) and in 2016 (the year the intervention was initiated, when all the high-risk patients were "randomized" to the intervention). An expanded set of features that included not only structured EMR data, but also NLP data extracted from clinical notes, geocode data linked to zip codes, and individual-level public records data extracted from commercial sources, could be used as predictors in the analysis. Difference-in-difference before-after comparison analysis could be used by combining patients above the intervention threshold with an equal or greater number of patients just slightly below the threshold in order to adjust for possible time trends. To the extent that prescriptive ML analysis shows that some high-risk VHA patients do not profit from the current REACH VET intervention, more intensive interventions could be targeted to patients with this profile in future implementations. It might even be possible to use a group-randomized (by treatment center) design (Treweek and Zwarenstein 2009) to assign the high-risk VHA patients predicted not to be helped by the current REACH VET intervention to different high-intensity evidence-based interventions designed specifically to treat suicidal patients, such as Dialectical Behavior Therapy, Cognitive Therapy for Suicide Prevention, or Collaborative Assessment and Management of Suicidality. This design would allow a more refined prescriptive ML analysis subsequently to be carried out to create a clinical decision support tool that helped clinicians implement precision treatment planning for high-risk VHA patients.

5.10 Conclusions

Improvements are needed in both the big data and the ML methods used to analyze these data if the full potential of ML is to be realized in addressing the suicide problem. It is likely that the prediction accuracy of the ML models reviewed here could be improved, perhaps substantially so, at low cost by more nuanced EMR feature transformation and by expanding the features to include information extracted from clinical notes using NLP and, in the US, from public data sources using zip code links (small area geocode data) and from commercially aggregated individual-level public records. Even better prediction is likely in health plans that routinely screen patients with self-reports of various sort (e.g., periodic completion of a self-report depression scale; Louzon et al. 2016; Simon et al. 2013). The ML analysis methods used in existing suicide prediction studies could also be improved substantially by using recently-developed ensemble and AutoML methods that optimize feature transformation-pruning, hyperparameter tuning, and adjustments for extreme imbalance in the outcome. Further work is needed to determine sample sizes at which such ML approaches are effective, especially for outcomes as rare as suicide.

We have no way of knowing how much suicide prediction accuracy would be improved by implementing all these feature expansions and ML analysis improvements, but it is almost certain that prediction accuracy would be insufficient to allow treatment planning to be based on such a model. Rather than use this fact, as critics have, to reject structured suicide risk assessment out of hand, it makes much more sense to see this phase of ML analysis as a useful first step in a multi-step process of need and risk evaluation. It is not inconceivable that SP in such an improved total-population first-stage ML model would be very close to 1.0 below a threshold that included a substantial proportion of patients. If so, it might be practical to ask all patients above that low-risk threshold to complete a structured self-report suicide risk assessment that included the full range of scales and performance-based neurocognitive tests that have been found to predict suicidal behavior in previous studies. A second-stage ML analysis in that subsample could then be carried out that used the predictors from the prior total-population analysis and the self-report measures obtained in the structured risk assessment to target the subset of patients who would receive an in-depth clinical suicide risk evaluation. The information in the self-report battery could be used as a starting point for this evaluation in the service of developing a treatment plan. A third-stage ML clinical decision support model based on input from all three predictor sets (i.e., the EMR data and other passive data available in the total-population, the structured patient self-report data available in the subsamples defined by the first ML model, and the clinical data collected in the smaller subgroup targeted by the second ML model) could then be developed to provide clinical decision support for this treatment planning. Part of the treatment process might then involve the use of new technologies supported by additional ML analyses, such as pharmacogenomics screening to select optimal medications (El-Mallakh et al. 2016) and use of new technologies to monitor ongoing treatment response as well as imminent suicide risk (Vahabzadeh et al. 2016). This kind of nested use of successively more refined ML models in which structured data are combined with clinical evaluations is likely to hold the key to maximizing the value of big data ML analysis in improving detection and treatment of suicidal patients.

References

Accurint (2018) http://www.accurint.com. Accessed 20 Feb 2018

Ahmedani BK, Simon GE, Stewart C, Beck A, Waitzfelder BE, Rossom R et al (2014) Health care contacts in the year before suicide death. J Gen Intern Med 29(6):870–877. https://doi.org/10.1007/s11606-014-2767-3

Barak-Corren Y, Castro VM, Javitt S, Hoffnagle AG, Dai Y, Perlis RH et al (2017) Predicting suicidal behavior from longitudinal electronic health records. Am J Psychiatry 174(2):154–162. https://doi.org/10.1176/appi.ajp.2016.16010077

Barros J, Morales S, Echávarri O, García A, Ortega J, Asahi T et al (2017) Suicide detection in Chile: proposing a predictive model for suicide risk in a clinical sample of patients with mood disorders. Rev Bras Psiquiatr 39:1–11

Beck AT, Steer RA (1988) BHS, Beck Hopelessness Scale: manual. Psychological Corporation, San Antonio

Beck AT, Schuyler D, Herman I (1974) Development of suicidal intent scales. In: Beck AT, Lettieri DJ, HLP R, National Institute of Mental Health, Center for Studies of Suicide Prevention, University of Pennsylvania Department of Psychiatry (eds) The prediction of suicide. Charles Press, Bowie, pp 45–56

Beck AT, Steer RA, Brown G (1996) Manual for the Beck Depression Inventory-II. Psychological Corporation, San Antonio

Ben-Ari A, Hammond K (2015) Text mining the EMR for modeling and predicting suicidal behavior among US veterans of the 1991 Persian gulf war. In: Paper presented at the 2015 48th Hawaii international conference on system sciences, 5–8 Jan 2015, pp 3168–3175. https://doi.org/10.1109/hicss.2015.382

Berman AL, Silverman MM (2014) Suicide risk assessment and risk formulation part II: suicide risk formulation and the determination of levels of risk. Suicide Life Threat Behav 44(4):432–443. https://doi.org/10.1111/sltb.12067

Bernert RA, Hom MA, Roberts LW (2014) A review of multidisciplinary clinical practice guidelines in suicide prevention: toward an emerging standard in suicide risk assessment and management, training and practice. Acad Psychiatry 38(5):585–592. https://doi.org/10.1007/s40596-014-0180-1

Bilen K, Ponzer S, Ottosson C, Castren M, Pettersson H (2013) Deliberate self-harm patients in the emergency department: who will repeat and who will not? Validation and development of clinical decision rules. Emerg Med J 30(8):650–656. https://doi.org/10.1136/emermed-2012-201235

Bolton JM (2015) Suicide risk assessment in the emergency department: out of the darkness. Depress Anxiety 32(2):73–75. https://doi.org/10.1002/da.22320

Bolton JM, Gunnell D, Turecki G (2015) Suicide risk assessment and intervention in people with mental illness. BMJ 351:h4978

Braithwaite SR, Giraud-Carrier C, West J, Barnes MD, Hanson CL (2016) Validating machine learning algorithms for twitter data against established measures of suicidality. JMIR Ment Health 3(2):e21. https://doi.org/10.2196/mental.4822

Brown JL, Swartzendruber A, DiClemente RJ (2013) Application of audio computer-assisted self-interviews to collect self-reported health data: an overview. Caries Res 47(Suppl 1):40–45. https://doi.org/10.1159/000351827

Bryan CJ, Rudd DM, Wertenberger E, Etienne N, Ray-Sannerud BN, Morrow CE et al (2014) Improving the detection and prediction of suicidal behavior among military personnel by measuring suicidal beliefs: an evaluation of the suicide cognitions scale. J Affect Disord 159:15–22. https://doi.org/10.1016/j.jad.2014.02.021

Carroll R, Metcalfe C, Gunnell D (2014) Hospital presenting self-harm and risk of fatal and non-fatal repetition: systematic review and meta-analysis. PLoS One 9(2):e89944. https://doi.org/10.1371/journal.pone.0089944

Carter G, Milner A, McGill K, Pirkis J, Kapur N, Spittal MJ (2017) Predicting suicidal behaviours using clinical instruments: systematic review and meta-analysis of positive predictive values for risk scales. Br J Psychiatry 210(6):387–395. https://doi.org/10.1192/bjp.bp.116.182717

Chawla N (2010) Data mining for imbalanced datasets: an overview. In: Maimon O, Rokach L (eds) Data mining and knowledge discovery handbook, 2nd edn. Springer, Berlin, pp 875–886

Chan MK, Bhatti H, Meader N, Stockton S, Evans J, O'Connor RC et al (2016) Predicting suicide following self-harm: systematic review of risk factors and risk scales. Br J Psychiatry 209(4):277–283. https://doi.org/10.1192/bjp.bp.115.170050

Choi SB, Lee W, Yoon JH, Won JU, Kim DW (2018) Ten-year prediction of suicide death using Cox regression and machine learning in a nationwide retrospective cohort study in South Korea. J Affect Disord 231:8–14. https://doi.org/10.1016/j.jad.2018.01.019

Chung DT, Ryan CJ, Hadzi-Pavlovic D, Singh SP, Stanton C, Large MM (2017) Suicide rates after discharge from psychiatric facilities: a systematic review and meta-analysis. JAMA Psychiat 74(7):694–702. https://doi.org/10.1001/jamapsychiatry.2017.1044

Cohen ZD, DeRubeis RJ (2018) Treatment selection in depression. Annu Rev Clin Psychol. https://doi.org/10.1146/annurev-clinpsy-050817-084746

Cook BL, Progovac AM, Chen P, Mullin B, Hou S, Baca-Garcia E (2016) Novel use of natural language processing (NLP) to predict suicidal ideation and psychiatric symptoms in a text-based mental health intervention in Madrid. Comput Math Methods Med 2016:8708434. https://doi.org/10.1155/2016/8708434

Cooper J, Kapur N, Dunning J, Guthrie E, Appleby L, Mackway-Jones K (2006) A clinical tool for assessing risk after self-harm. Ann Emerg Med 48(4):459–466. https://doi.org/10.1016/j.annemergmed.2006.07.944

Cooper J, Steeg S, Bennewith O, Lowe M, Gunnell D, House A et al (2013) Are hospital services for self-harm getting better? An observational study examining management, service provision and temporal trends in England. BMJ Open 3(11):e003444. https://doi.org/10.1136/bmjopen-2013-003444

Dhingra K, Boduszek D, O'Connor RC (2015) Differentiating suicide attempters from suicide ideators using the integrated motivational-volitional model of suicidal behaviour. J Affect Disord 186:211–218. https://doi.org/10.1016/j.jad.2015.07.007

Dickerson F, Adamos M, Katsafanas E, Khushalani S, Origoni A, Savage C et al (2017) The association between immune markers and recent suicide attempts in patients with serious mental illness: a pilot study. Psychiatry Res 255:8–12. https://doi.org/10.1016/j.psychres.2017.05.005

El-Mallakh RS, Roberts RJ, El-Mallakh PL, Findlay LJ, Reynolds KK (2016) Pharmacogenomics in psychiatric practice. Clin Lab Med 36(3):507–523. https://doi.org/10.1016/j.cll.2016.05.001

Feurer M, Klein A, Eggensperger K, Springenberg JT, Blum M, Hutter F (2015) Efficient and robust automated machine learning. Paper presented at the proceedings of the 28th International Conference on Neural Information Processing Systems - volume 2, Montreal, Canada, 2015

Franklin JC, Ribeiro JD, Fox KR, Bentley KH, Kleiman EM, Huang X et al (2017) Risk factors for suicidal thoughts and behaviors: a meta-analysis of 50 years of research. Psychol Bull 143(2):187–232. https://doi.org/10.1037/bul0000084

Glenn CR, Nock MK (2014) Improving the short-term prediction of suicidal behavior. Am J Prev Med 47(3 Suppl 2):S176–S180. https://doi.org/10.1016/j.amepre.2014.06.004

Gnambs T, Kaspar K (2015) Disclosure of sensitive behaviors across self-administered survey modes: a meta-analysis. Behav Res Methods 47(4):1237–1259. https://doi.org/10.3758/s13428-014-0533-4

Greist JH, Gustafson DH, Stauss FF, Rowse GL, Laughren TP, Chiles JA (1973) A computer interview for suicide-risk prediction. Am J Psychiatry 130(12):1327–1332. https://doi.org/10.1176/ajp.130.12.1327

Greist JH, Mundt JC, Gwaltney CJ, Jefferson JW, Posner K (2014) Predictive value of baseline electronic Columbia-Suicide Severity Rating Scale (eC-SSRS) assessments for identifying risk of prospective reports of suicidal behavior during research participation. Innov Clin Neurosci 11(9–10):23–31

He H, Garcia EA (2009) Learning from imbalanced data. IEEE Trans Knowl Data Eng 21(9):1263–1284. https://doi.org/10.1109/tkde.2008.239

Hettige NC, Nguyen TB, Yuan C, Rajakulendran T, Baddour J, Bhagwat N et al (2017) Classification of suicide attempters in schizophrenia using sociocultural and clinical features: a machine learning approach. Gen Hosp Psychiatry 47:20–28. https://doi.org/10.1016/j.genhosppsych.2017.03.001

Holtkamp CR, Weaver RC (2018) Quantifying the relationship between social capital and economic conditions in Appalachia. Appl Geogr 90:175–186. https://doi.org/10.1016/j.apgeog.2017.12.010

Hunter C, Chantler K, Kapur N, Cooper J (2013) Service user perspectives on psychosocial assessment following self-harm and its impact on further help-seeking: a qualitative study. J Affect Disord 145(3):315–323. https://doi.org/10.1016/j.jad.2012.08.009

Ilgen MA, Downing K, Zivin K, Hoggatt KJ, Kim HM, Ganoczy D et al (2009) Exploratory data mining analysis identifying subgroups of patients with depression who are at high risk for suicide. J Clin Psychiatry 70(11):1495–1500. https://doi.org/10.4088/JCP.08m04795

Jobes DA, Au JS, Siegelman A (2015) Psychological approaches to suicide treatment and prevention. Curr Treat Options Psychiatry 2(4):363–370. https://doi.org/10.1007/s40501-015-0064-3

Jobes DA, Comtois KA, Gutierrez PM, Brenner LA, Huh D, Chalker SA et al (2017) A randomized controlled trial of the collaborative assessment and management of suicidality versus enhanced care as usual with suicidal soldiers. Psychiatry 80(4):339–356. https://doi.org/10.1080/00332747.2017.1354607

Joiner TE Jr, Buchman-Schmitt JM, Chu C (2017) Do undiagnosed suicide decedents have symptoms of a mental disorder? J Clin Psychol 73(12):1744–1752. https://doi.org/10.1002/jclp.22498

Jordan P, Shedden-Mora MC, Lowe B (2018) Predicting suicidal ideation in primary care: an approach to identify easily assessable key variables. Gen Hosp Psychiatry 51:106–111. https://doi.org/10.1016/j.genhosppsych.2018.02.002

Just MA, Pan L, Cherkassky VL, McMakin D, Cha C, Nock MK et al (2017) Machine learning of neural representations of suicide and emotion concepts identifies suicidal youth. Nat Hum Behav 1:911–919. https://doi.org/10.1038/s41562-017-0234-y

Katz C, Bolton J, Sareen J (2016) The prevalence rates of suicide are likely underestimated worldwide: why it matters. Soc Psychiatry Psychiatr Epidemiol 51(1):125–127. https://doi.org/10.1007/s00127-015-1158-3

Katz C, Randall JR, Sareen J, Chateau D, Walld R, Leslie WD et al (2017) Predicting suicide with the SAD PERSONS scale. Depress Anxiety 34(9):809–816. https://doi.org/10.1002/da.22632

Kessler RC (2018) The potential of predictive analytics to provide clinical decision support in depression treatment planning. Curr Opin Psychiatry 31(1):32–39. https://doi.org/10.1097/yco.0000000000000377

Kessler RC, Warner CH, Ivany C, Petukhova MV, Rose S, Bromet EJ et al (2015) Predicting suicides after psychiatric hospitalization in US Army soldiers: the Army Study to Assess Risk and Resilience in Servicemembers (Army STARRS). JAMA Psychiat 72(1):49–57. https://doi.org/10.1001/jamapsychiatry.2014.1754

Kessler RC, Hwang I, Hoffmire CA, McCarthy JF, Petukhova MV, Rosellini AJ et al (2017a) Developing a practical suicide risk prediction model for targeting high-risk patients in the veterans health administration. Int J Methods Psychiatr Res 26(3). https://doi.org/10.1002/mpr.1575

Kessler RC, Stein MB, Petukhova MV, Bliese P, Bossarte RM, Bromet EJ et al (2017b) Predicting suicides after outpatient mental health visits in the Army Study to Assess Risk and Resilience in Servicemembers (Army STARRS). Mol Psychiatry 22(4):544–551. https://doi.org/10.1038/mp.2016.110

Koldsland BO, Mehlum L, Mellesdal LS, Walby FA, Diep LM (2012) The suicide assessment scale: psychometric properties of a Norwegian language version. BMC Res Notes 5:417. https://doi.org/10.1186/1756-0500-5-417

Kreitman N, Foster J (1991) The construction and selection of predictive scales, with special reference to parasuicide. Br J Psychiatry 159:185–192

Large M, Myles N, Myles H, Corderoy A, Weiser M, Davidson M et al (2017a) Suicide risk assessment among psychiatric inpatients: a systematic review and meta-analysis of high-risk categories. Psychol Med 48(7):1119–1127. https://doi.org/10.1017/s0033291717002537

Large MM, Ryan CJ, Carter G, Kapur N (2017b) Can we usefully stratify patients according to suicide risk? BMJ 359:j4627

Larkin C, Di Blasi Z, Arensman E (2014) Risk factors for repetition of self-harm: a systematic review of prospective hospital-based studies. PLoS One 9(1):e84282. https://doi.org/10.1371/journal.pone.0084282

Levine S, Ancill RJ, Roberts AP (1989) Assessment of suicide risk by computer-delivered self-rating questionnaire: preliminary findings. Acta Psychiatr Scand 80(3):216–220

Lindqvist D, Nimeus A, Traskman-Bendz L (2007) Suicidal intent and psychiatric symptoms among inpatient suicide attempters. Nord J Psychiatry 61(1):27–32. https://doi.org/10.1080/08039480601122064

Linehan MM, Korslund KE, Harned MS, Gallop RJ, Lungu A, Neacsiu AD et al (2015) Dialectical behavior therapy for high suicide risk in individuals with borderline personality disorder: a randomized clinical trial and component analysis. JAMA Psychiat 72(5):475–482. https://doi.org/10.1001/jamapsychiatry.2014.3039

Louzon SA, Bossarte R, McCarthy JF, Katz IR (2016) Does suicidal ideation as measured by the PHQ-9 predict suicide among VA patients? Psychiatr Serv 67(5):517–522. https://doi.org/10.1176/appi.ps.201500149

Luedtke AR, van der Laan MJ (2016) Optimal individualized treatments in resource-limited settings. Int J Biostat 12(1):283–303. https://doi.org/10.1515/ijb-2015-0007

Luoma JB, Martin CE, Pearson JL (2002) Contact with mental health and primary care providers before suicide: a review of the evidence. Am J Psychiatry 159(6):909–916. https://doi.org/10.1176/appi.ajp.159.6.909

Madsen T, Erlangsen A, Nordentoft M (2017) Risk estimates and risk factors related to psychiatric inpatient suicide-an overview. Int J Environ Res Public Health 14(3). https://doi.org/10.3390/ijerph14030253

McCarthy JF, Bossarte R, Katz IR, Thompson C, Kemp J, Hannemann C et al (2015) Predictive modeling and concentration of the risk of suicide: implications for preventive interventions in the US Department of Veterans Affairs. Am J Pub Health 105(9):1935–1942. https://doi.org/10.2105/AJPH.2015.302737

McCoy TH Jr, Castro VM, Roberson AM, Snapper LA, Perlis RH (2016) Improving prediction of suicide and accidental death after discharge from general hospitals with natural language processing. JAMA Psychiatry 73(10):1064–1071. https://doi.org/10.1001/jamapsychiatry.2016.2172

Mulder R, Newton-Howes G, Coid JW (2016) The futility of risk prediction in psychiatry. Br J Psychiatry 209(4):271–272. https://doi.org/10.1192/bjp.bp.116.184960

Murphy GE (1972) Clinical identification of suicidal risk. Arch Gen Psychiatry 27:356–359

National Institute for Health and Care Excellence (NICE) (2011) Self-harm in over 8s: long-term management. //www.nice.org.uk/guidance/cg133. Accessed 5 Jan 2018

Nock MK, Park JM, Finn CT, Deliberto TL, Dour HJ, Banaji MR (2010) Measuring the suicidal mind: implicit cognition predicts suicidal behavior. Psychol Sci 21(4):511–517. https://doi.org/10.1177/0956797610364762

Nordt C, Warnke I, Seifritz E, Kawohl W (2015) Modelling suicide and unemployment: a longitudinal analysis covering 63 countries, 2000-11. Lancet Psychiatry 2(3):239–245. https://doi.org/10.1016/s2215-0366(14)00118-7

O'Connor E, Gaynes BN, Burda BU, Soh C, Whitlock EP (2013) Screening for and treatment of suicide risk relevant to primary care: a systematic review for the U.S. Preventive Services Task Force. Ann Intern Med 158(10):741–754. https://doi.org/10.7326/0003-4819-158-10-201305210-00642

Oh J, Yun K, Hwang JH, Chae JH (2017) Classification of suicide attempts through a machine learning algorithm based on multiple systemic psychiatric scales. Front Psych 8:192. https://doi.org/10.3389/fpsyt.2017.00192

Olfson M, Marcus SC, Bridge JA (2014) Focusing suicide prevention on periods of high risk. JAMA 311(11):1107–1108. https://doi.org/10.1001/jama.2014.501

Olson RS, Sipper M, La Cava W, Tartarone S, Vitale S, Fu W et al. (2017) A system for accessible artificial intelligence. arXiv.org. arXiv:1705.00594v2

Owens D, Kelley R (2017) Predictive properties of risk assessment instruments following self-harm. Br J Psychiatry 210(6):384–386. https://doi.org/10.1192/bjp.bp.116.196253

Owens C, Hansford L, Sharkey S, Ford T (2016) Needs and fears of young people presenting at accident and emergency department following an act of self-harm: secondary analysis of qualitative data. Br J Psychiatry 208(3):286–291. https://doi.org/10.1192/bjp.bp.113.141242

Palmer L, Blackwell H, Strevens P (2007) Service users' experience of emergency services following self harm: a national survey of 509 patients. College Centre for Quality Improvement, Royal College of Psychiatrists. https://www.rcpsych.ac.uk/pdf/National%20SU%20Survey%20Final%20Self%20Harm%20Project.pdf. Accessed 20 Feb 2018

Passos IC, Mwangi B, Cao B, Hamilton JE, Wu MJ, Zhang XY et al (2016) Identifying a clinical signature of suicidality among patients with mood disorders: a pilot study using a machine learning approach. J Affect Disord 193:109–116. https://doi.org/10.1016/j.jad.2015.12.066

Patterson WM, Dohn HH, Bird J, Patterson GA (1983) Evaluation of suicidal patients: the SAD PERSONS scale. Psychosomatics 24(4):343–345, 348–349. https://doi.org/10.1016/s0033-3182(83)73213-5

Pearson A, Saini P, Da Cruz D, Miles C, While D, Swinson N et al (2009) Primary care contact prior to suicide in individuals with mental illness. Br J Gen Pract 59(568):825–832. https://doi.org/10.3399/bjgp09X472881

Pestian JP, Sorter M, Connolly B, Cohen KB, McCullumsmith C, Gee JT et al (2017) A machine learning approach to identifying the thought markers of suicidal subjects: a prospective multicenter trial. Suicide Life Threat Behav 47(1):112–121. https://doi.org/10.1111/sltb.12312

Polley E, LeDell E, van der Laan M (2016) SuperLearner: Super learner prediction [computer program]. R package version 2.0–21: The Comprehensive R Archive Network

Posner K, Brown GK, Stanley B, Brent DA, Yershova KV, Oquendo MA et al (2011) The Columbia-Suicide Severity Rating Scale: initial validity and internal consistency findings from three multisite studies with adolescents and adults. Am J Psychiatry 168(12):1266–1277. https://doi.org/10.1176/appi.ajp.2011.10111704

Poulin C, Shiner B, Thompson P, Vepstas L, Young-Xu Y, Goertzel B et al (2014) Predicting the risk of suicide by analyzing the text of clinical notes. PLoS One 9(1):e85733. https://doi.org/10.1371/journal.pone.0085733

Quinlivan L, Cooper J, Steeg S, Davies L, Hawton K, Gunnell D et al (2014) Scales for predicting risk following self-harm: an observational study in 32 hospitals in England. BMJ Open 4(5):e004732. https://doi.org/10.1136/bmjopen-2013-004732

Quinlivan L, Cooper J, Davies L, Hawton K, Gunnell D, Kapur N (2016) Which are the most useful scales for predicting repeat self-harm? A systematic review evaluating risk scales using measures of diagnostic accuracy. BMJ Open 6(2):e009297. https://doi.org/10.1136/bmjopen-2015-009297

Quinlivan L, Cooper J, Meehan D, Longson D, Potokar J, Hulme T et al (2017) Predictive accuracy of risk scales following self-harm: multicentre, prospective cohort study. Br J Psychiatry 210(6):429–436. https://doi.org/10.1192/bjp.bp.116.189993

Randall JR, Rowe BH, Dong KA, Nock MK, Colman I (2013) Assessment of self-harm risk using implicit thoughts. Psychol Assess 25(3):714–721. https://doi.org/10.1037/a0032391

Reutfors J, Brandt L, Ekbom A, Isacsson G, Sparen P, Osby U (2010) Suicide and hospitalization for mental disorders in Sweden: a population-based case-control study. J Psychiatr Res 44(12):741–747. https://doi.org/10.1016/j.jpsychires.2010.02.003

Rosen A (1954) Detection of suicidal patients: an example of some limitations in the prediction of infrequent events. J Consult Psychol 18(6):397–403

Rudd MD (2014) Core competencies, warning signs, and a framework for suicide risk assessment in clinical practice. In: Nock MK (ed) The Oxford handbook of suicide and self-injury, 1st edn. Oxford University Press, Cary, pp 323–336. https://doi.org/10.1093/oxfordhb/9780195388565.013.0018

Rudd MD, Bryan CJ, Wertenberger EG, Peterson AL, Young-McCaughan S, Mintz J et al (2015) Brief cognitive-behavioral therapy effects on post-treatment suicide attempts in a military sample: results of a randomized clinical trial with 2-year follow-up. Am J Psychiatry 172(5):441–449. https://doi.org/10.1176/appi.ajp.2014.14070843

Runeson B, Odeberg J, Pettersson A, Edbom T, Jildevik Adamsson I, Waern M (2017) Instruments for the assessment of suicide risk: a systematic review evaluating the certainty of the evidence. PLoS One 12(7):e0180292. https://doi.org/10.1371/journal.pone.0180292

Schaffer A, Sinyor M, Kurdyak P, Vigod S, Sareen J, Reis C et al (2016) Population-based analysis of health care contacts among suicide decedents: identifying opportunities for more targeted suicide prevention strategies. World Psychiatry 15(2):135–145. https://doi.org/10.1002/wps.20321

Silverman JJ, Galanter M, Jackson-Triche M, Jacobs DG, Lomax JW, Riba MB et al (2015) The American Psychiatric Association practice guidelines for the psychiatric evaluation of adults. Am J Psychiatry 172(8):798–802. https://doi.org/10.1176/appi.ajp.2015.1720501

Simon GE, Rutter CM, Peterson D, Oliver M, Whiteside U, Operskalski B et al (2013) Does response on the PHQ-9 Depression Questionnaire predict subsequent suicide attempt or suicide death? Psychiatr Serv 64(12):1195–1202. https://doi.org/10.1176/appi.ps.201200587

Spittal MJ, Pirkis J, Miller M, Carter G, Studdert DM (2014) The Repeated Episodes of Self-Harm (RESH) score: a tool for predicting risk of future episodes of self-harm by hospital patients. J Affect Disord 161:36–42. https://doi.org/10.1016/j.jad.2014.02.032

Steeg S, Kapur N, Webb R, Applegate E, Stewart SL, Hawton K et al (2012) The development of a population-level clinical screening tool for self-harm repetition and suicide: the ReACT self-harm rule. Psychol Med 42(11):2383–2394. https://doi.org/10.1017/s0033291712000347

Stefansson J, Nordstrom P, Runeson B, Asberg M, Jokinen J (2015) Combining the Suicide Intent Scale and the Karolinska Interactive Violence Scale in suicide risk assessments. BMC Psychiatry 15:226. https://doi.org/10.1186/s12888-015-0607-6

Steinberg D, Phillip C (1997) CART – classification and regresstion trees. Salford Systems, San Diego

Taylor TL, Hawton K, Fortune S, Kapur N (2009) Attitudes towards clinical services among people who self-harm: systematic review. Br J Psychiatry 194(2):104–110. https://doi.org/10.1192/bjp.bp.107.046425

Tran T, Luo W, Phung D, Harvey R, Berk M, Kennedy RL et al (2014) Risk stratification using data from electronic medical records better predicts suicide risks than clinician assessments. BMC Psychiatry 14:76. https://doi.org/10.1186/1471-244x-14-76

Treweek S, Zwarenstein M (2009) Making trials matter: pragmatic and explanatory trials and the problem of applicability. Trials 10:37. https://doi.org/10.1186/1745-6215-10-37

Urbanowicz RJ, Meeker M, Lacava W, Olson RS, Moore JH (2017) Relief based feature selection: introduction and review. arXiv.org. arXiv:1711.08421

VA Office of Inspector General (2007) Health care inspection: impementing VHA's mental health strategic plan initiatives for suicide prevention. https://www.va.gov/oig/54/reports/VAOIG-06-03706-126.pdf

VA Office of Public and Intergovernmental Affairs (2017) VA REACH VET initiative helps save veterans lives: program signals when more help is needed for at-risk veterans. U.S. Department of Veterans Affairs. https://www.va.gov/opa/pressrel/pressrelease.cfm?id=2878. Accessed 12 May 2017

Vahabzadeh A, Sahin N, Kalali A (2016) Digital suicide prevention: can technology become a game-changer? Innov Clin Neurosci 13(5–6):16–20

VanderWeele TJ, Leudtke AR, van der Laan MJ, Kessler RC (2018) Selecting optimal subgroups for treatment using many covariates. arXiv.org. arXiv:1802.09642

Vermeulen K, Vansteelandt S (2015) Bias-reduced doubly robust estimation. J Am Stat Assoc 110(511):1024–1036. https://doi.org/10.1080/01621459.2014.958155

Walsh G, Sara G, Ryan CJ, Large M (2015) Meta-analysis of suicide rates among psychiatric in-patients. Acta Psychiatr Scand 131(3):174–184. https://doi.org/10.1111/acps.12383

Walsh CG, Ribeiro JD, Franklin JC (2017) Predicting risk of suicide attempts over time through machine learning. Clin Psychol Sci 5(3):457–469. https://doi.org/10.1177/2167702617691560

Wilkinson ST, Sanacora G (2016) Ketamine: a potential rapid-acting antisuicidal agent? Depress Anxiety 33(8):711–717. https://doi.org/10.1002/da.22498

Woodford R, Spittal MJ, Milner A, McGill K, Kapur N, Pirkis J et al (2017) Accuracy of clinician predictions of future self-harm: a systematic review and meta-analysis of predictive studies. Suicide Life Threat Behav. https://doi.org/10.1111/sltb.12395

World Health Organization (WHO) (2018a) Mental health: suicide data. http://www.who.int/mental_health/prevention/suicide/suicideprevent/en/. Accessed 20 Feb 2018

World Health Organization (WHO) (2018b) Age-standardized suicide rates (per 100 000 population), 2015. Global Health Observatory (GHO) data. http://www.who.int/gho/mental_health/suicide_rates/en/. Accessed 03 Mar 2018

Emerging Shifts in Neuroimaging Data Analysis in the Era of "Big Data"

6

Danilo Bzdok, Marc-Andre Schulz, and Martin Lindquist

Advances in positron emission tomography (PET) and functional magnetic resonance imaging (fMRI) have revolutionized our understanding of human cognition and its neurobiological basis. However, a modern imaging setup often costs several million dollars and requires highly trained technicians to conduct data acquisition. Brain-imaging studies are typically laborious in logistics and data management, and require costly-to-maintain infrastructure. The often small numbers of scanned participants per study have precluded the deployment of and potential benefits from advanced statistical methods in neuroimaging that tend to require more data (Bzdok and Yeo 2017; Efron and Hastie 2016). In this chapter we discuss how the increased information granularity of burgeoning neuroimaging data repositories—in both number of participants and measured variables per participant—will motivate and require new statistical approaches in everyday data analysis. We put particular emphasis on the implications for the future of precision psychiatry, where brain-imaging has the potential to improve diagnosis, risk detection, and treatment choice by clinical-endpoint prediction in single patients. We argue that the statistical properties of approaches tailored for the data-rich setting promise improved clinical translation of empirically justified single-patient prediction in a fast, cost-effective, and pragmatic manner.

D. Bzdok (✉)
Department of Psychiatry and Psychotherapy, RWTH Aachen University, Aachen, Germany

Jülich Aachen Research Alliance (JARA)—Translational Brain Medicine, Aachen, Germany

Parietal Team, INRIA, Gif-sur-Yvette, France
e-mail: danilo.bzdok@rwth-aachen.de

M.-A. Schulz
Department of Psychiatry and Psychotherapy, RWTH Aachen University, Aachen, Germany

M. Lindquist
Department of Biostatistics, Johns Hopkins University, Baltimore, MD, USA

I. C. Passos et al., *Personalized Psychiatry*,
https://doi.org/10.1007/978-3-030-03553-2_6

6.1 Blessing and Curse of Increasing Information Content in Neuroimaging

The notion of "big data" in modern neuroimaging arises in two related, yet importantly different ways. On the one hand, the number of observed variables per participant, called "feature dimensionality" (p) and, on the other hand, the available "sample size" (n) of scanned participants. In traditional experimental studies in psychology, neuroscience, and medicine the number of observed variables has rarely exceeded the number of participants. Concretely, many common neuropsychological questionnaires and medical assessments capture <30 items—few in comparison to the often hundreds of participants in clinical trials. This so-called "long-data" setting (participants n > variables p) is the realm of classical statistics. Around the turn of the century, the development of whole-genome sequencing and brain-imaging led to biology and medicine entering the high-dimensional, or "wide-data", setting (variables p >> participants n; Efron 2012; Efron and Hastie 2016). For example, in genetics, the feature dimensionality from the ~3 billion base pairs or the >100,000 single nucleotide polymorphisms summarizing the human genome vastly exceeds the size of typically collected participant cohorts.

The brain sciences have recently been argued to be the most data-rich among all medical specialties (Nature Editorial 2016). A single brain scan with high-resolution MRI can easily exceed 100,000 variables that collectively describe brain morphology or a type of neural activity. However, over the last 20 years, the sample size in a typical brain-imaging study has rarely exceeded 50–100 participants. We argue that important statistical consequences arise from the divergence of the "n-p ratio" (the relation between the number of participants and the number of variables per observation) in the classical and high-dimensional settings.

High-resolution MRI increases the potential for new neurobiological findings, but the increased information detail in the brain recordings also exacerbates the dangers of the so-called "curse of dimensionality" (Bellman 1957; Friedman et al. 2001). Humans are accustomed to operating in the physical world and our geometric perception is fine-tuned to 3-dimensional environments. Human intuition regarding geometric properties, such as volume or distance, tends to struggle and eventually go awry in high-dimensional spaces. Mathematically, an increase in feature dimensionality (imagine going from a line to a square to a cube) leads to an exponential increase in the input-data space, and the available data points become increasingly sparse so that even the volumetric brain scans of monozygotic twins may look dissimilar in high dimensions. In brain-imaging, an increase in resolution (such as more voxels or more scans per time) will offer more detailed information, but the higher information granularity will also make the relevant neurobiological structure more difficult to identify. With respect to the brain data themselves, this volume increase entails that, with each (uncorrelated) new variable, investigators would potentially need to scan exponentially more participants to populate the input variable space at the same density (Bishop 2006). With respect to machine learning algorithms applied to brain data, it means that with more input variables per participant, a pattern-recognition algorithm will increasingly struggle to find interesting statistical relations that exist in the data. The considerable increase in data abundance and complexity will put many classical statistical methods at risk of being deemed obsolete, and replaced by modeling approaches better tailored to the new data reality in imaging neuroscience.

6.2 Recent Trends for Data Collection and Collaboration Across Laboratories

The acquisition of brain-imaging data at scale is a challenging undertaking due to a variety of technical, logistic, and legal factors. These hurdles range from the need for time-effective and harmonized measurement protocols, to the participants' informed consent for sharing their data. New brain-imaging projects have tackled many of these challenges and aim to provide general-purpose datasets to the neuroscientific and psychiatric research community. Here, we give an overview of the current state of "big-data" brain-imaging, and illustrate important ramifications for data-analysis practices due to the increasing data accumulation.

Three data initiatives stand out in the brain-imaging landscape (Smith and Nichols 2018): The Human Connectome Project (HCP), the UK Biobank (UKBB) Imaging Study, and the Enhancing NeuroImaging Genetics through Meta-Analysis (ENIGMA) Consortium. The HCP, launched 2009, was one of the earliest attempts to create a rich reference dataset for the brain-imaging community. As the name suggests, an important goal of the HCP initiative was to promote insight into functional connectivity architecture by providing extensive multimodal data on a large number of healthy participants. The HCP consortium recently completed multi-modal measurements of over 1200 healthy adults (aged 22–35), including 300 twin pairs. For each participant, the project gathered structural, functional, and diffusion MRI, genotyping data, as well as a large variety (>400) of demographic, behavioral, and lifestyle indicators. With genetic profiling and extensive phenotyping with several thousand descriptors, UKBB is even more comprehensive. This data collection initiative set out in 2006 to gather genetic and environmental (e.g., nutrition, lifestyle, medications) data from 500,000 volunteers, and is currently the world's largest biomedical dataset. UKBB recruited adults between the ages of 40 and 69. The participants will be followed for >25 years, including repeated measurements and access to their electronic health records. In 2014 UKBB launched its brain-imaging extension, aiming to gather structural, functional, diffusion, and susceptibility-weighted MRI of 100,000 participants by 2022 (Miller et al. 2016). Yet another ambitious attempt to create a large-scale neuroimaging dataset is the ENIGMA consortium, launched in 2009. Compared to UKBB and HCP, ENIGMA takes a different approach by centrally coordinating research projects and providing each participating group with analysis pipelines and quality control protocols. The software is run independently by each acquisition site and the ensuing results are combined into integrative summary analyses, possibly across different imaging modalities (i.e. structural, functional, or diffusion MRI). Because of this, the sample size can be on the order of several thousand participants depending on the availability of brain-scans directly relevant for a particular research question.

In sum, we portrayed three contemporary data-aggregation projects, which have substantially different research agendas. While UKBB is above all a medical dataset and was designed for large-scale population epidemiology, the ambition of HCP lies in functional and anatomical connectivity in healthy subjects, whereas ENIGMA has an important emphasis on genetic profiling in combination with brain scanning. Many more comparable datasets are in the making and should, within the next decade, multiply the amount of brain imaging data available for research.

Compared to many traditional MRI experiments consisting of only a few dozen participants, large-scale projects such as HCP and UKBB have unprecedented strengths and pave the way for new neuroscientific insights. A key aspect is the study design. Most imaging studies have a *retrospective* or *cross-sectional* nature in that the investigators first decide what they are looking for (e.g., a certain disease diagnosis or behavioral facet), and then recruit participants that fulfill the inclusion criteria. The phenotype of interest has already been identified, and the study is in some sense looking into the past. In contrast, UKBB is a *prospective* epidemiological study. A broad sample of the population is included in the expectation that a relevant set of the participants will experience a variety of health-relevant events at some point in the future. For example, among the 100,000 participants to be brain-scanned, ~1800 are expected to develop Alzheimer's disease by 2022, ~8000 will develop diabetes, ~1800 will have experienced a stroke, and ~1200 will be affected by Parkinson's disease (Sudlow et al. 2015). Once these medical conditions have developed, data will be available to the investigators consisting of information before, and on the path to, disease onset. This potentially unprecedented wealth of longitudinal information can be leveraged to identify early disease markers and new risk factors; perhaps even chart hypotheses that might not have occurred to researchers when designing a retrospective study. As most diseases only develop in a small percentage of the population, sampling a large number of participants is necessary for prospective studies to gain traction. Such future-oriented data aggregation designs have great potential for early disease detection and trans-diagnostic stratification in mental health.

Despite much enthusiasm, the creation, curation, and collaboration of extensive brain-imaging datasets also raise a series of technical challenges (Arbabshirani et al. 2017; Bzdok and Meyer-Lindenberg 2018; Woo et al. 2017). Inter-scanner differences and the need for quality control at scale come into play. Effective data collection is complicated by the fact that brain-imaging is highly sensitive to differences in scanner type and configuration. For example, scanner-specific differences in the measured longitudinal changes in regional gray matter volume emerge even for identical scanner models (Takao et al. 2013). Multi-site data collection projects should take into consideration that these inter-scanner differences can confound statistical analysis (Focke et al. 2011). Reducing the heterogeneity of the acquired data is either costly (i.e., requires multiple identical setups), or reduces collection efficiency (i.e., single-scanner bottleneck). Different existing projects make different trade-offs between collection efficiency and incurred inter-scanner effects. ENIGMA prioritizes collection efficiency by working in parallel on a variety of different types of scanners. To minimize confounding influences due to inter-scanner effects, UKBB uses identical scanner hardware at the different acquisition sites, while the HCP has relied on a single scanner for the entirety of their data acquisition.

Moreover, common quality control procedures that are usually performed by hand can become infeasible. Undetected technical artifacts, movement artifacts, or human error in applying the measurement protocol can distort statistical analysis. In traditional small- to medium-scale studies, even in HCP, it was still possible to perform quality control manually. A researcher or technician could visually inspect the data for each participant and scanning modality to check for errors and artifacts. The sheer amount of brain data that is generated in large-scale brain-imaging projects makes the manual approach to quality control overly time-consuming. UKBB has conceived and implemented automated quality control procedures (Alfaro-Almagro et al. 2018). This approach uses pattern-learning algorithms to model the data distribution and automatically identify artifacts and measurement errors. UKBB, HCP, and ENIGMA have invested in elaborate automated processing pipelines and protocols to detect and correct errors and guarantee standardized data.

6.3 Anticipating Upcoming Shifts in Statistical Practice

Once successfully collected and controlled for quality, massive brain-imaging datasets allow for more ambitious statistical analyses than standard studies consisting of only a few dozen participants. Recently, more advanced statistical and computational approaches have emerged to address new research goals, such as the search for neuroimaging biomarkers and hidden brain phenotypes that are demonstrated to be useful at the single-subject level. We will discuss in detail four key directions in which the increased amount of data in brain-imaging is likely to usher in changes to everyday statistical data-analysis practice. We anticipate, first, a trend for parametric methods to be complemented by flexible non-parametric methods that allow for more detailed models of the brain. Second, a trend for discriminative methods to be complemented by more applications of generative models that aim to uncover the mechanisms for how the observed data arose. Third, a tendency for frequentist and Bayesian approaches to be combined for data analysis solutions that are both computationally cheap and holistic in interpretation. Fourth, out-of-sample generalization will become an increasingly attractive alternative to classical null-hypothesis hypothesis testing. Below, we discuss each direction in turn. We will also describe how "big-data" innovations can potentially aid in the analysis at the single-subject level, providing a mechanism for precision psychiatry.

An important benefit of large-scale data collection is that it allows for more *expressive* models for describing phenomena in the brain—models that can capture higher-order non-linear interactions in the data and are able to represent more subtle aspects about the brain (i.e., increased model expressiveness). There are two ways in which this can happen. First, increased participant sample sizes make it possible to extract details and nuances from the data distribution that would be indistinguishable from random fluctuations in small studies. Second, more data points allow for a higher number of parameters to be reliably estimated, allowing for more expressive models that can instantiate more complicated neural phenomena (i.e., models that can reproduce potentially extremely complex statistical relationships; Devroye et al. 1996; Bickel and Doksum 2007).

Classical statistical methods, such as *t*-test, analysis of variance (ANOVA), and linear regression, used for example in the widely distributed statistical parametric mapping (SPM) software package, do not exhibit the properties necessary for representing increasingly complicated brain properties with an increasing number of participants. Classical methods attempt to model data with a fixed, limited number of parameters, and usually make rigid assumptions about the underlying structure of the brain measurements. For example, the *t*-test and ANOVA usually assume Gaussianity regardless of the underlying data distribution observed in the MRI brain scans. After accumulating enough participants to detect a statistically significant effect, additional data may yield little additional insights. In fact, classical methods may frequently underfit the data in more complex data settings with many input variables. The use of a fixed number of parameters qualifies these methods as *parametric*. In contrast, *non-parametric* approaches (Fig. 6.1) typically make weaker assumptions about the underlying structure of the acquired brain data. Here the number of parameters can flexibly adapt with the number of participants, and is potentially infinite. Data from more participants allow for more nuanced quantitative brain representations, based on less rigid statistical models.

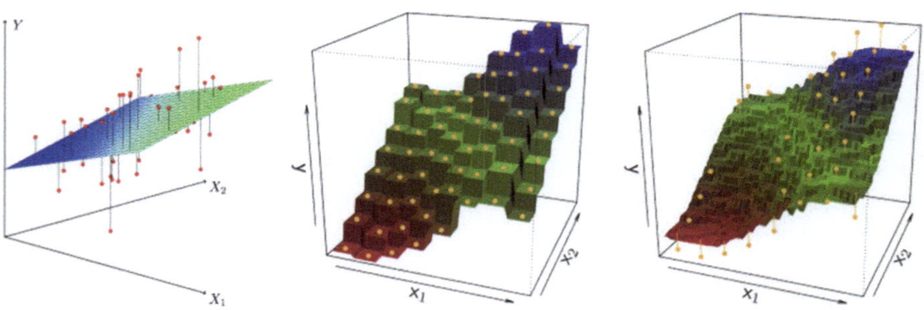

Fig. 6.1 *Parametric vs. non-parametric approaches.* Non-parametric methods (with a number of parameters that scales with increasing data availability) are more flexible than parametric methods (with a fixed number of parameters). We illustrate this distinction for the case of predicting a target variable Y based on two input variables X_1 and X_2. The parametric method of linear regression (left) always estimates three parameters defining the plane that best explains variation in the data. The number of parameters is independent of the number of data points and independent of the shape in which the data points are distributed—the end result is always a plane. In contrast, the non-parametric k-nearest-neighbor algorithm (middle and right) can adapt to a more complex shape by increasing the number of parameters in step with the number of available data points. With ample amount of available data points (right, $k = 9$), the shape of the regression surface turns from a coarse step function (middle, $k = 1$) into a smooth approximation of the data distribution (right). Non-parametric methods adapt their number of parameters in step with the number of data points and can thus reproduce more complex shapes and distributions. Reproduced from James et al. (2013)

An example of a non-parametric method is the *k*-nearest neighbor algorithm (Fig. 6.1). A sample (e.g., a T1 image of a healthy or schizophrenic participant) is classified by the class membership (disease status) of the majority of its closest data points in the dataset (the other participants). As the number of samples increase, more details of the data distribution (e.g., individual brain anatomy) can be captured leading to a more refined quantitative representation of the brain phenomenon under study. Other popular examples of non-parametric methods are decision trees (and tree-based methods such as random forests) and kernel support vector machines. In both approaches the number of model parameters scales naturally with the number of participants. Extensive biomedical datasets are ideal for using non-parametric methods to capture previously unobserved neurobiological properties that might be ignored when using parametric methods alone.

An example of the application of non-parametric methods in brain-imaging is the investigation by Gennatas et al. (2017) on how gray-matter changes with age in a large neurodevelopmental dataset (Pennsylvania Neurodevelopmental Cohort, 1189 participants aged 8 to 23). A parametric approach would have been to use an instance of the (parametric) generalized linear model (GLM) to relate MRI gray-matter measures to age, that is to estimate coefficients for the variables (gray-matter measures) that best predict the target (age). Instead, Gennatas and colleagues used a non-parametric extension of the GLM called "generalized additive models" (GAM; Hastie and Tibshirani 1990). Instead of fitting a coefficient for each input variable, GAMs estimate an adaptive functional form linking each individual variable with the respective output variable. With more data points (participants), the identified arbitrarily complex input-output functions could more accurately reflect the interaction between gray matter voxels and overall participant age. The GAM is thus able to describe and exploit highly non-linear statistical relationships to which the GLM would be blind[1]. Integrating the non-linear relationships between regional gray-matter volumes and age increased the goodness of fit of the model, leading to less noisy parameter estimates and therefore to enhanced understanding of gray-matter changes in individual brain regions across the lifespan.

As a second important distinction, statistical models can be used to address a research goal directly—discriminative models—or additionally learn intrinsic structure from the data at hand—generative models (Fig. 6.2). As an analogy, assume somebody wants to distinguish between speech from Japanese and Chinese speakers. A generative model would first try to learn the grammar, vocabulary, and phonology of both languages. Only then would the model address the classification-goal of disambiguating whether a certain speaker is Japanese or Chinese based on an explicit internal representation of what each of the two languages looks like. A discriminative model, on the other hand, would use any aspect of the speech, such as the intonation or the frequency of certain phoneme combinations, to somewhat blindly distinguish the speaker groups—even if no deeper understanding is obtained

[1]The only way for the GLM to describe non-linear interactions is to anticipate the particular effect and introduce the corresponding higher-order terms explicitly into GLM model from the beginning.

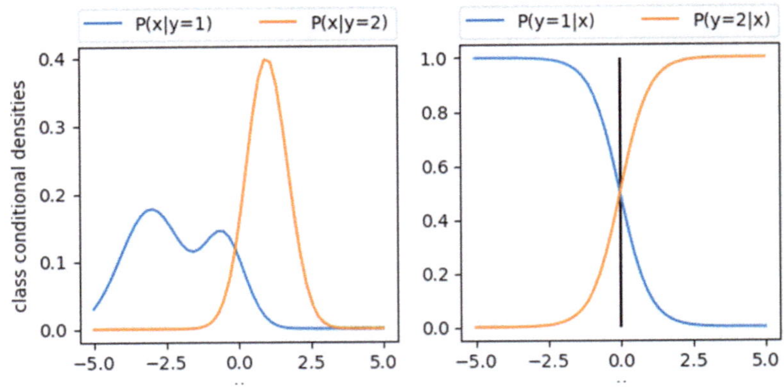

Fig. 6.2 *Generative vs. discriminative approaches.* Patients (black) and controls (red) both undergo the same biomedical evaluation. The result of the test is indicated on the x-axis, the likelihood that a participant of either class will receive a particular result is indicated on the y-axis (left). There exist two statistical approaches to predict if a given participant is patient or control based on the test result. A discriminative model (right) estimates a decision boundary (vertical line) that optimally separates the patients from the controls. Apart from the decision boundary, no other information is extracted from the data. A generative model (left) estimates the full probability distributions of both the patient and control group. The probability distributions are then used to determine whether a given participant is more likely to be patient or control. The generative model also captures information about the data distribution that does not directly help to distinguish patients from controls (e.g., information about the far ends of the probability distributions or about the density bump at $x = -1$). This "unnecessary" information can reveal important biological insights: In this case, the density bump at $x = -1$ could indicate that the patient group is in fact composed of two different groups with distinct symptom profiles. Inspired by Murphy (2012)

about the speech's content and structure. In a large number of application domains in empirical research, discriminative models have dominated statistical analysis. In the example of distinguishing[2] a healthy group from a schizophrenic patient group, discriminative models (e.g., logistic regression, support vector machines) learn a decision boundary between the participants from each group (think of a dividing line between categories, e.g., healthy vs. diseased)—or, more formally, they estimate the posterior probability[3] $P(y|x)$, without extracting an explicit representation of each class to be distinguished. In contrast, generative models (e.g., naive Bayes classifier) estimate the joint distribution $P(x,y)$—or, more informally, generative

[2]The classification setting serves as an illustration only. Discriminative methods exist independently of the classification—regression divide. For example, the clustering algorithm k-means is discriminative in the sense that it finds decision boundaries between clusters, although it attempts neither classification nor regression.

[3]$P(y|x)$ is the so-called conditional (in the Bayesian terminology the "posterior") probability: The probability of an event y (e.g., the patient is diseased) under the condition that another event x (e.g., a certain brain anatomy measured by MRI) has already occurred. $P(x,y)$ is the so called joint probability: The probability of x and y occurring together.

methods model the process by which the data was generated (Jebara 2012; Bishop and Lasserre 2007). The class posterior distributions $P(y|x)$ can then be derived using Bayes' rule.

Importantly, generative models have the intrinsic ability to produce new, artificial data samples. This ability to create never-observed data that is characteristic for one of the classes has an appealing advantage. Sampling from the generative model and visually inspecting the generated samples can provide direct insights into the inner workings of the brain phenomenon under study. In a model of the brain, where one model parameter is hypothesized to represent age, varying this parameter would allow the investigator to see a brain aging before their eyes—providing insight into age-related brain changes. However, a natural caveat is that the results will only be as good as the underlying model. If the model does not accurately depict the phenomena in question, the output of a generative model will be similarly flawed.

As a consequence, generative models are usually easier to interpret than most discriminative models because the modeled internal representation of what the data "looks like" (i.e., the conditional variation between input variables, output variables, and possible hidden variables) has been noted to capture biologically meaningful structure in previous brain-imaging studies. Furthermore, many generative models work by adaptively modeling hidden states of a system, or by finding a compact set of hidden factors that describe the dynamics of the system at hand. This process is often called *latent factor* discovery (Goodfellow et al. 2016, Chap. 13). A compact set of latent factors is usually easier to interpret than potentially high-dimensional brain-imaging input data (Fig. 6.3). A simple example of such a latent factor based generative model is the commonly used independent component analysis (ICA). ICA reduces the data to a manageable number of hidden directions of variation. As a generative model, ICA is able to produce never observed, artificial data samples based on the extracted latent factors. Such sources of variation underlying the observations can be easily interpreted (e.g., by plotting which brain areas associated with which latent factor) and can uncover previously unknown information about the brain in both health and disease. Given enough samples of resting-state fMRI time series, ICA is able to both find hidden multivariate patterns that together explain the variation in the data (e.g., the default mode network) and generate new artificial brain images from the derived factors. The combined statistical goal of generative methods to model hidden states of the brain phenomena and minimize an optimization criterion at hand (e.g., prediction performance) is usually more challenging than the statistical goal of discriminative models to simply find a decision boundary between classes. This explains why generative models tend to require brain data from more participants and why they are now becoming increasingly attractive with large-scale datasets.

A common generative model in brain-imaging is dynamic causal modeling (DCM) invented by Friston et al. (2003). The goal of DCM is to estimate directed "effective connectivity", that is, the functional influence that one brain region exerts on another brain region. DCM explicitly estimates interactions between neuronal populations in the context of a biophysical model of the hemodynamic response. This characteristic makes DCM a generative model with neurobiological plausibility

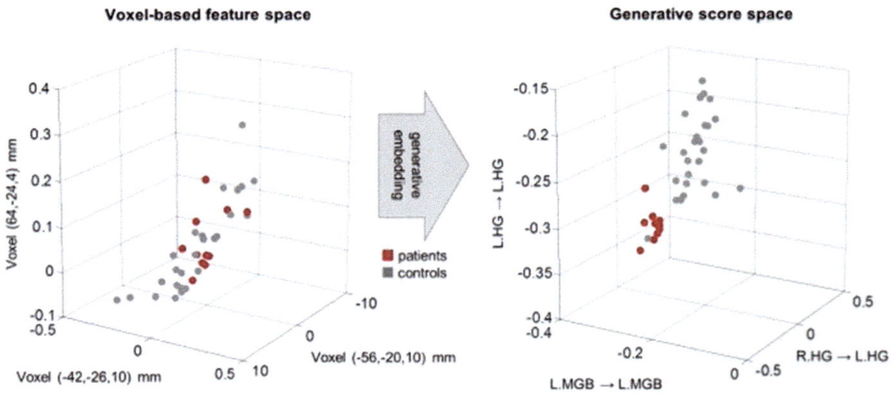

Fig. 6.3 *Latent factor model in action.* Dynamic causal modeling is a brain-imaging analysis technique that can be used to model the functional connectivity in the brain. DCM uses fMRI activity data to estimate the degree of connectedness between predefined brain regions. The DCM model parameters can be seen as a different perspective on the same data: Each participant has different fMRI activity and thus different estimated DCM model parameters. Here, whole-brain fMRI data do not lend themselves to distinguish patients from controls. The figure on the left shows how patients and controls are distributed in the space spanned by three voxels ("voxel-based feature space"). The DCM parameters capture more meaningful biological concepts than individual voxels, and patients and controls become separable. The figure on the right shows how participants form clusters of patients and controls when viewed in the space spanned by three DCM connectivity parameters ("generative score space"). Reproduced from Brodersen et al. (2011)

that is able to synthesize plausible hemodynamic activation patterns from hidden neural activity in brain regions. In addition to various human fMRI studies, the plausibility of DCM has been directly evidenced in rats by successfully relating intracerebral EEG recordings to rat fMRI (David et al. 2008).

It should be noted that not every generative model is based on latent factor discovery, and not every latent factor model qualifies as a generative model. Some generative approaches work by transforming random input vectors (e.g., generative adversarial networks) or autoregressive models (e.g., pixelRNN, waveNet) and do not lend themselves to easy introspection of the underlying statistical relationships by the investigator. An example of a non-generative latent factor model is classical canonical correlation analysis[4] (CCA). This exploratory method is similar to principal component analysis in that it reduces the data to orthogonal principal vectors, but instead of maximizing explained variance, CCA maximizes the correlation between two (lower-dimensional) latent factors of two data "views", for example, brain-imaging on the one hand and behavioral performance scores on the other hand. CCA thus identifies aspects of brain-imaging data and behavioral data that exhibit maximal linear correspondence with each other.

[4]Although there exists a generative probabilistic variant of CCA, the widely used classical CCA is not inherently generative.

For instance, Wang et al. (2018) used canonical correlation analysis to provide some of the first evidence for distinct neurobiological underpinnings of different subjective experiences of mind-wandering. Such stimulus-independent cognitive processes are associated, amongst others, with executive performance and creativity indicators. To provide evidence that mind-wandering is not a homogeneous psychological construct, but instead comprises a range of cognitive architectures and functions, the authors employed CCA with resting-state fMRI data as one view and self-reported experience, cognitive performance, and psychological well-being data as the other view. The CCA revealed latent factors that simultaneously described individual variation in self-reported experience and connectivity in the default mode network, as well as factors uniquely related to aspects of cognition, such as executive control and creativity. These findings, enabled by the unique modeling capabilities of CCA, provided evidence that distinct brain dimensions collectively contribute to different cognitive aspects underlying the mind-wandering experience.

Traditionally, perhaps the most important distinction in statistics in general and in neuroimaging in particular has been between *frequentist* and *Bayesian* models (Freedman 1995). To illustrate, let us consider the example of medical research. A Bayesian researcher would happily introduce prior knowledge from past research and experience into her statistical inferences to guide further upcoming research. These a-priori assumptions placed on the model parameters in combination with Bayes' rule yield full probability distributions, that is, a point estimate and detailed information on the uncertainty that comes with, for example, the effectiveness of the proposed treatment. The frequentist medical researcher, on the other hand, would shy away from the subjectivity of making a-priori assumptions before studying the data. She obtains an estimate without detailed uncertainty information—for the treatment effectiveness that hold with fewer assumptions about the underlying data-generating process. Intuitively, Bayesian statistics is a good choice for several research questions being asked using neuroimaging techniques. Commonly accepted knowledge of brain anatomy and physiology can for instance be used as a basis to come up with a-priori assumptions that guide the model fitting process. In the example of DCM, interactions between neuronal populations are modeled not just based on the experimental data, but instead the modeling process is couched in probabilistic a-priori knowledge concerning hemodynamic parameters, anatomical regions, and more.

In contrast to many approaches to full Bayesian inference, performing statistical data analysis using a frequentist approach is usually computationally cheaper (Bishop and Lasserre 2007; Jordan 2011; Yang et al. 2016). The "model evidence" term in Bayes' formula is typically the source of the much increased computational load in the Bayesian setting. It is an integral over all possible values of all relevant parameters (which are often much more numerous than the feature dimensionality of the actual quantitative observations in the brain) that usually cannot be directly solved, and even reaching approximate solutions is computationally challenging in many cases. A common tool for these approximations, the family of Markov chain Monte Carlo (MCMC) methods, is an iterative algorithm that is not easily parallelizable. These hurdles become even more severe in domains such as brain-imaging, where an arms race for increasingly finer spatial and temporal resolution is constantly pushing the feature dimensionality of the brain scans. One potential solution to the computational expense of Bayesian inference in many applications to extensive brain data is the integration of Bayesian and frequentist modeling paradigms. An example of such a hybrid approach is variational inference—a widespread modeling solution to approximate complicated Bayesian integrals (Jordan et al. 1999). Another hybrid approach that has been shown effective is *shrinkage*, a statistical estimation method in which individual observations "borrow strength" from a larger group of observations (Bzdok et al. 2017; Varoquaux et al. 2010; Mejia et al. 2015). Shrinkage is implicit in Bayesian inference, penalized likelihood inference, and multi-level models and is directly related to the empirical Bayes estimators commonly used in neuroimaging (Friston et al. 2002; Friston and Penny 2003).

A combined Bayesian-frequentist approach was also applied by Brodersen et al. (2011) in the aim of computational psychiatry. Faced with the challenge of classifying a small number of participants into healthy and diseased groups based on the high-dimensional input data from all voxel activities in the whole fMRI time series, they introduced classification via "generative embeddings". These investigators used Bayesian, generative dynamic causal modeling to compute effective-connectivity models for each participant. The DCM model parameters were then used as a low-dimensional effective summary of the high-dimensional voxel data (Fig. 6.3). This dimensionality reduction via domain knowledge (i.e., priors on brain anatomy and physiology in the DCM) mitigated the curse of dimensionality and, in a subsequent step of the modeling approach, allowed for the data to be classified by a frequentist support vector machine, thereby combining the strengths of both Bayesian and frequentist inference.

Finally, in mainstream statistics as routinely applied in medicine, psychology, and brain-imaging, new knowledge is typically derived from data by means of *null-hypothesis testing*, that is testing whether or not an observation is too extreme to be plausible under the null-hypothesis of no effect (Fisher and Mackenzie 1923; Neyman and Pearson 1933). In a drug trial, the null-hypothesis would be that the new drug is no more effective than a current standard treatment. A measured effectiveness that defies explanation as a random fluctuation in the experiment would lead the investigator to discard the null-hypothesis and establish the superiority of the new drug. An overarching theme of classical statistics in the twentieth century was to optimally exploit small sample sizes using low-dimensional parametric models (Efron and Hastie 2016).

The recent advent of large-scale data collection has had two important consequences. First, caveats emerge for hypothesis testing in ever more high-dimensional neuroimaging data. The "multiple comparisons" problem becomes increasingly challenging to address in the wide-data scenario (Miller 1981; Efron 2012). The traditional approach in the brain-imaging community is called "mass univariate" analysis and performs separate statistical tests for each brain location. When many null-hypothesis tests are being carried out in concert, an increasing number of false positive findings will plague the data analysis and subsequent interpretation. Many commonly used methods to explicitly account for the number of false positives, such as Bonferroni's method for family-wise error correction, work by increasing the threshold for statistical significance in a conservative fashion, which substantially increases the number of participants whose brain data are necessary to reject a given null-hypothesis.

On the other hand, if the number of variables is small (e.g., after reducing whole-brain data to a lower-dimension using independent component analysis) but the number of participants happens to be much larger, even very small, practically irrelevant statistical effects will sooner or later become significant (Berkson 1938). For instance, brain-behavior correlations of $r \approx 0.1$ were consistently found to be statistically significant when considering a sample of $n = 5000$ participants even after correction for multiple comparisons (Miller et al. 2016). This and similar examples illustrate that, in the era of "big-data" neuroimaging, hypothesis testing may more and more often struggle to distinguish between statistical and practical significance. In sum, the traditional null-hypothesis testing frameworks may have to tackle new difficulties in analysis settings with a lot of input variables ("wide-data" or $n << p$ setting) and when brain data from a large human population are considered ("long-data" or $n > p$ setting).

At the same time, the rise of national, continental, and intercontinental brain-data collections are making the statistical goal of prediction increasingly attractive. Modern machine-learning approaches have a focus on predicting disease status, behavior, even treatment response of single individuals. The process of deriving new knowledge based on a sample of participants takes a different form in the predictive analysis setting. Instead of looking within the sample of participants at the properties of the estimated parameters, the focus is on accurate statements about *new*, previously unseen participants—and evaluating the *out-of-sample generalization* (Vapnik 1998; Valiant 1984). In practice, the participants are split into two groups: a "training set" that is used to fit the model or classifier, and a separate "test set" that is used to evaluate prediction performance. If the prediction succeeds on the test set, we can empirically establish that the model captures useful biological structure and, more importantly, that a meaningful connection between (potentially many) input variables (e.g., fMRI brain scans) and a target variable (e.g., disease status) exists. Usually, the random split into train- and test-set is performed repeatedly in a procedure that is called *cross-validation*.

By quantifying the prediction success in new individuals (i.e., out-of-sample estimates) many machine learning approaches naturally adopt a prospective viewpoint and can directly yield a notion of clinical relevance. In contrast, classical approaches based on null-hypothesis testing often take a retrospective flavor as they usually revolve around finding statistical effects in the dataset at hand (so-called in-sample estimates) based on prespecified modeling assumptions, typically without explicitly evaluating some fitted models on unseen or future data points. Hence, ubiquitous techniques for out-of-sample generalization in machine learning are likely candidates for enabling a future of personalized psychiatry. This is because predictive models can be applied to and obtain answers from a single patient.

Two properties are shared between the discussed upcoming trends in data-analysis in the brain-imaging community. On the one hand, the anticipated shifts in statistical practice are expected to enable more complex (e.g., increased model expressiveness) and also more interpretable statistical models (e.g., more generative models) of the brain, based on high-dimensional neuroimaging data. On the other hand, many of these modeling approaches tend to work better with larger participant sample sizes and may be well prepared to handle rich high-dimensional input data. With the advent of the new data reality in the brain-imaging community, such "data-hungry" methods become increasingly feasible and necessary.

6.4 Clinical Endpoint Prediction in Single Psychiatric Patients Based on Brain-Imaging

In this last section, we place the trends of large-scale data collection and ensuing changes in statistical practice in the context of current mental health research. We give examples of how large-scale neuroimaging datasets can enable new research approaches and use a recent paper by Drysdale et al. (2017) to illustrate how parametric structure-discovery methods, latent factor models, and out-of-sample prediction all can be integrated in this type of research agenda.

The traditional approach to mental health research consists of identifying symptoms that frequently occur together and using these clinical manifestations to define disease-specific symptom combinations based on expert opinion. Clusters of symptoms are assumed to define coherent disease entities. These disease definitions are then used to find diagnostic biomarkers (e.g., by searching for neural correlates) or to predict treatment response. While this approach has worked well in many areas of medicine (consider, for example, the glomerular filtration rate to identify kidney disease) the same success has not yet materialized in psychiatry. Brain-based quantitative markers for predicting treatment response at the single-subject level, even to reliably distinguish between disease subtypes or healthy and diseased participants, remain elusive in mental health (Insel and Cuthbert 2015). Large-scale brain-imaging allows for flipping this approach on its head. Instead of clustering individuals into groups by clinical symptoms and then looking for neurophysiological correlates, we can cluster based on quantitative brain measurements directly (letting the brain data "speak for themselves") and then look at symptom measurements and clinical endpoints only after identifying clusters of shared brain dysfunction. As this alternative strategy underlies the ambition to directly model the biological basis of the disease and is less vulnerable to subjective and overlapping symptoms, it may be more likely to yield a reliable foundation for diagnosis and treatment.

Depression is one of many cases in psychiatry where recent evidence emphasizes unclear correspondence between diagnostic labels used in clinical practice and their neurobiological substrates as elucidated in neuroscientific research. Drysdale and colleagues employ functional neuroimaging to identify depression subtypes in brain biology (Fig. 6.4). In a large-scale study ($n = 1188$) they identified patterns of functional connectivity in resting-state fMRI that were associated with symptoms

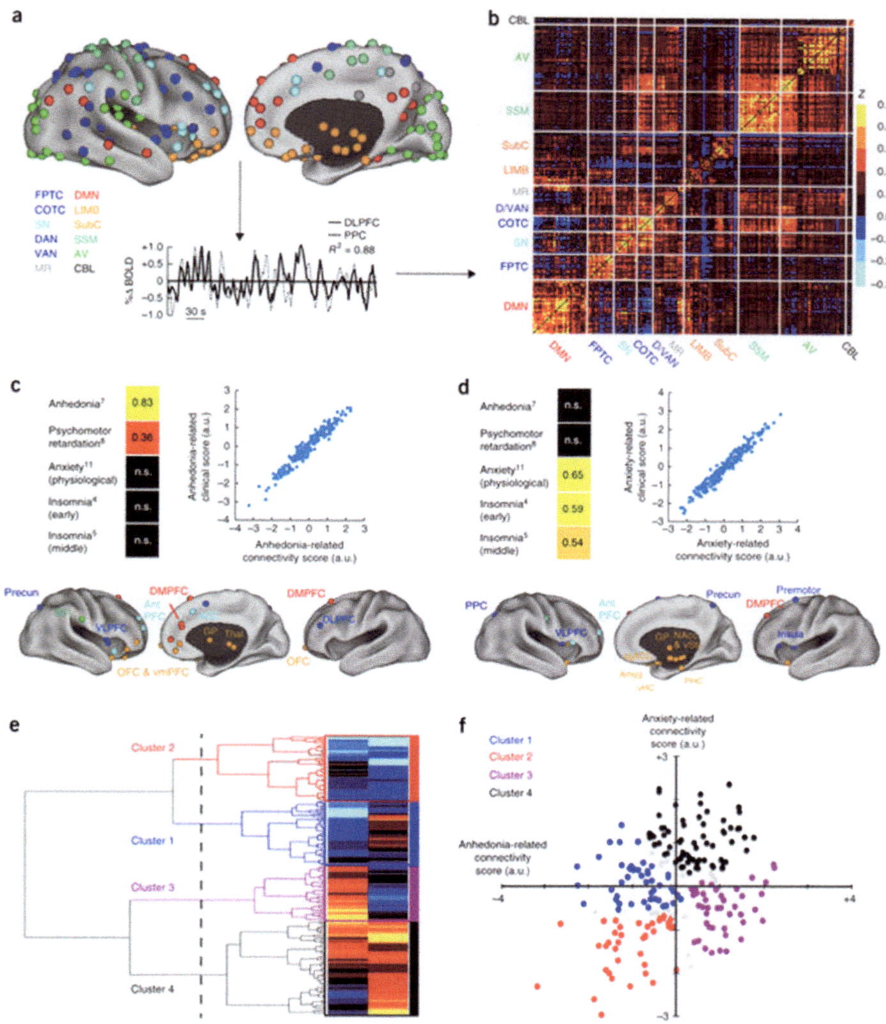

Fig. 6.4 *Example of modern brain-imaging-based subject stratification.* Neural activity time series measured by fMRI were extracted from regions of interest (**a**) and correlated with each other to yield "functional connectivity features" (**b**). Canonical correlation analysis was then used to find a small set of linear combinations of functional connectivity features that are maximally correlated with self-reported symptoms of depression (**c**, **d**). Thus, the number of variables per participant was reduced by two preparation steps: First from whole-brain maps to region-wise activity measures, then from functional connectivity features to even fewer components of variation obtained from CCA. This dimensionality reduction of high-resolution imaging data allowed identifying clusters of participants (**e**, **f**) which are predictive of distinct symptom-profiles and response to transcranial magnetic stimulation treatment. Reproduced from Drysdale (2017)

of depression and used these to identify four neurobiologically distinct subtypes of depression ("biotypes"). Based on these alternative group distinction for depressed patients they were then able to predict whether or not a patient would respond to transcranial magnetic stimulation (TMS)—a therapy in which a pulsing magnetic field is used to induce inhibitory or excitatory electric current into parts of the brain. The analysis approach in this study consisted of three steps: First, the authors built a *latent factor* model connecting fMRI and depression symptoms via CCA. Second, they used *parametric, discriminative* clustering to identify subtypes based on the previously derived latent factors. Third, they used support vector machines as a discriminative classifier to achieve *out-of-sample* predictions for the depression subtype based on fMRI data.

To better illustrate how the statistical methods tie into the quest for depression biomarkers we will cover the analysis pipeline more comprehensively. After preprocessing (the cortex and subcortical structures were parcellated into 258 regions of interest), resting-state fMRI time series were extracted for each region and correlated against each other. The resulting correlation coefficients (functional connectivity features) for each patient represented the left-hand side of the variable set for a canonical correlation analysis. The right-hand side of the variable set was given by the corresponding Hamilton Depression Rating Scale results for each patient. The CCA then returned hidden dimensions of variation—sets of distinct functional connectivity patterns correlated with distinct combinations of clinical symptoms. The number of latent factors was much smaller than the number of original regions, making the latent modeling results easier to analyze and interpret. The latent variability components were then used for clustering via the parametric *k*-means algorithm. This procedure used the similarity in functional connectivity to partition participants into k group such that each participant belonged to the cluster with the smallest mean distance. A split into four clusters appeared to provide useful partitioning solutions for defining maximally dissimilar patient subtypes.

Each of these subtypes (i.e., clusters derived from the latent factors) was shown to be correlated both with distinct patterns of abnormal functional connectivity as well as distinct clinical-symptom profiles. All four subtypes also featured shared functional connectivity patterns that corresponded to "core" symptoms that were present in all patients diagnosed with depression. The individual subtype predicted whether or not a given patient would respond to transcranial magnetic stimulation therapy. Support vector machines were trained to directly predict a patient's brain-derived subtype based on their functional connectivity information.

The steps of the analysis pipeline (latent factor model, clustering, prediction) were conducted on a training data set consisting of only two-thirds of the patients, in order to be able to test how well the discovered brain-behavior effect is likely to generalize to previously "untouched" data (the remaining one-third). That is, the built support vector machines prediction models were validated on the previously held-out test set and achieved accuracy rates of approximately 90% in predicting the biological subtype of individual patients—and thereby their individual response to TMS treatment. This study is one of the first proofs of concept that data-derived brain phenotypes of psychiatric disorders can provide useful biological categories that enable improved treatment choices on a single-subject basis.

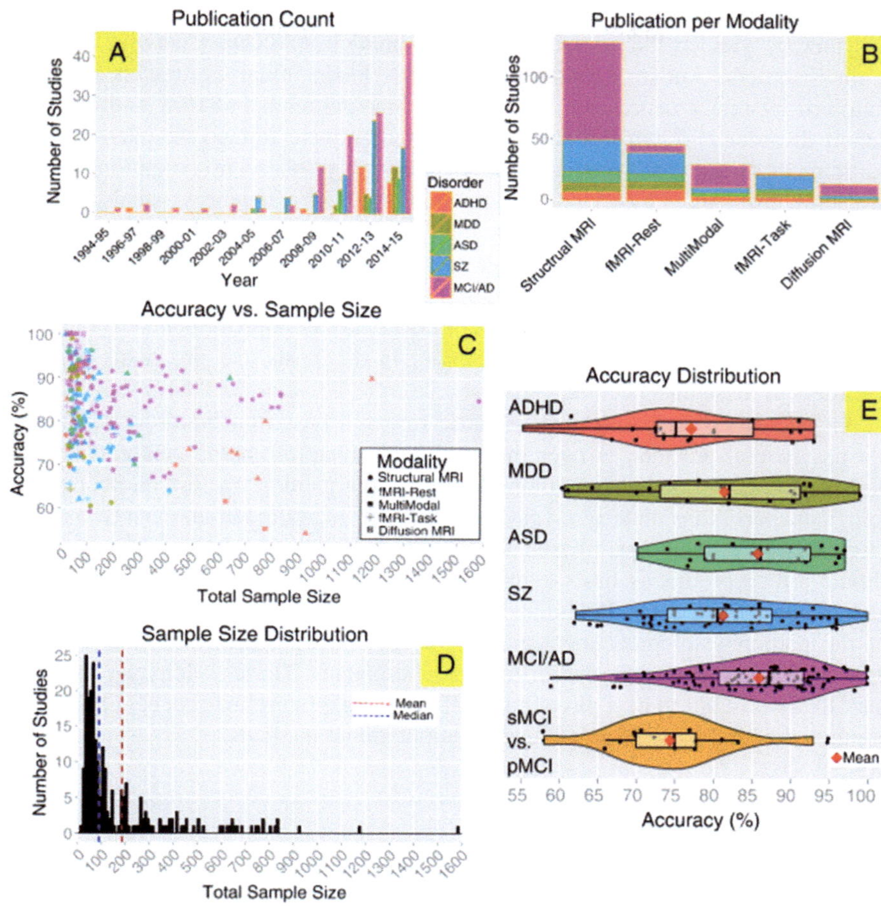

Fig. 6.5 *Single-subject prediction of brain disorders using neuroimaging.* A survey by Arbabshirani et al. (2017) shows strong growth in the number of brain-scanning studies that attempt to automatically classify brain disorders based on neuroimaging data (**a**). Structural MRI is so far the most frequently used input data for the purpose of classification (**b**). The number of participants is still relatively small (<200) for most imaging-based classification studies (**c**, **d**). Based on selected brain-imaging modalities and feature variables, different studies report diverging classification performances (**e**). Reproduced from Arbabshirani et al. (2017)

Over the last years, there has been a rising number of investigations into single-subject prediction of brain disorders in neuroimaging. Arbabshirani et al. (2017) recently provided a survey (Fig. 6.5) of ~200 recent studies. Based on their broad field analysis, structural and resting-state MRI are the brain-imaging modalities that are currently favored for predicting brain disorders, and most important brain disorders have been studied for single-subject prediction. Likely because of its severity and prevalence, mild cognitive impairment and Alzheimer's disease (MCD/AD) is the disorder that has most often been tried to predict based on

MRI data. The average prediction accuracy across studies was ~86% for MCD/AD and thereby yielded the comparatively best prediction accuracy among common brain disorders. Autism spectrum disorder yielded similar accuracies (~85%), followed by major depressive disorder and schizophrenia (~81%), and attention deficit disorder (~77%). Models in these studies were trained on relatively few participants (mean 186, median 88). Virtually all of these investigations had to restrict themselves to a correspondingly small number of features, usually derived by averaging brain regions via a brain atlas, or other biologically inspired manually crafted features. The reported average participant numbers were still an order of magnitude away from the projected number of (e.g., Alzheimer's) patients in the prospective UKBB study, leading us to anticipate further improvements in predictive accuracy and potential clinical applicability in diagnosis and prognosis of brain disorders as these data become available.

An intensified approach to psychiatric research based on brain-derived markers has several advantages over the traditional symptom-based research stream. Neuroimaging biomarkers can more directly allow gaining traction on neurophysiological aberrations underlying psychopathology. Identified brain-derived markers often enable reliable brain-based stratification of individual participants, which should offer a promising basis to improve clinical practice in diagnosis, prognosis, and treatment selection. Potential for more complete detection and exploitation of the pathophysiological mechanisms underlying brain disorders may fuel the development of new and superior treatment strategies. These anticipated advances may likely turn out to be a direct result of large-scale neuroimaging data collection combined with the use of data-hungry computational methods.

6.5 Conclusions

The soaring cost of psychiatric disease prompts a global urgency for finding new solutions (Bloom et al. 2012; Gustavsson et al. 2011). We believe that whether or not personalized medicine can be realized in psychiatry is largely a statistical question at its heart. For many decades, *the group* has served as the working unit of psychiatric research. Facilitated and intensified acquisition of always more detailed and diverse information on psychiatric patients is now bringing another working unit within reach—*the single patient*. Rather than pre-assuming disease categories and formally verifying prespecified neurobiological hypotheses, an increasingly attractive alternative goal is to let the data speak for themselves. As a consequence of the new data reality and changing research questions, some long trusted statistical methods may no longer be the best tool at our disposal.

The statistical properties of learning-algorithm approaches tailored for the data-rich setting promise clinical translation of empirically justified single-patient prediction in a fast, cost-effective, and pragmatic manner. Patient-level predictive analytics might also help psychiatry to move from strong reliance on symptom phenomenology to catch up with the biology-centered decision making in other branches of medicine. Machine learning tools offer an ideal data-guided framework to uncover, foster, and leverage inter-individual variation in behavior, brain, and genetics. The fact that the currently embraced mechanistic explanations for psychiatric disorders range from molecular histone-tail methylation in the cell nucleus to urbanization trends in society as a whole highlights human-independent learning algorithms as an underexploited avenue for the automatic identification of disease-specific neurobiological features that can predict clinical outcomes. Ultimately, the human intelligence alone may be insufficient to decipher how mental disorders arise at the complex interplay between each individual's unique genetic endowment and world experience.

References

Alfaro-Almagro F et al (2018) Image processing and quality control for the first 10,000 brain imaging datasets from UK Biobank. NeuroImage 166:400–424

Arbabshirani MR et al (2017) Single subject prediction of brain disorders in neuroimaging: promises and pitfalls. NeuroImage 145:137–165

Bellman R (1957) Dynamic programming. Princeton University Press, Princeton

Berkson J (1938) Some difficulties of interpretation encountered in the application of the chi-square test. J Am Stat Assoc 33(203):526–536

Bickel PJ, Doksum KA (2007) Mathematical statistics: basic ideas and selected topics. Pearson, Upper Saddle River

Bishop CM (2006) Machine learning and pattern recognition. Information science and statistics. Springer, Heidelberg

Bishop CM, Lasserre J (2007) Generative or discriminative? Getting the best of both worlds. Bayesian Stat 8(3):3–24

Bloom DE et al (2012) The global economic burden of noncommunicable diseases. No. 8712. Program on the global demography of aging

Brodersen KH et al (2011) Generative embedding for model-based classification of fMRI data. PLoS Comput Biol 7(6):e1002079

Bzdok D, Meyer-Lindenberg A (2018) Machine learning for precision psychiatry: opportunities and challenges. Biol Psychiatry Cogn Neurosci Neuroimaging 3(3):223–230

Bzdok D, Yeo BTT (2017) Inference in the age of big data: future perspectives on neuroscience. NeuroImage 155:549–564

Bzdok D, Eickenberg M, Varoquaux G, Thirion B (2017) Hierarchical region-network sparsity for high-dimensional inference in brain imaging. Inf Process Med Imaging 10265:323–335

David O et al (2008) Identifying neural drivers with functional MRI: an electrophysiological validation. PLoS Biol 6(12):2683–2697

Devroye L, Györfi L, Lugosi G (1996) A probabilistic theory of pattern recognition. Springer, New York

Drysdale AT et al (2017) Resting-state connectivity biomarkers define neurophysiological subtypes of depression. Nat Med 23(1):28–38

Editorial (2016) Daunting data. Nature 539:467–468

Efron B (2012) Large-scale inference: empirical Bayes methods for estimation, testing, and prediction. Cambridge University Press, Cambridge

Efron B, Hastie T (2016) Computer age statistical inference. Cambridge University Press, Cambridge

Fisher RA, Mackenzie WA (1923) Studies in crop variation. II. The manurial response of different potato varieties. J Agric Sci 13(3):311–320

Focke NK et al (2011) Multi-site voxel-based morphometry—not quite there yet. NeuroImage 56(3):1164–1170

Freedman D (1995) Some issues in the foundation of statistics. Found Sci 1(1):19–39
Friedman J, Hastie T, Tibshirani R (2001) The elements of statistical learning. Springer Series in Statistics, New York
Friston K, Penny W (2003) Posterior probability maps and SPMs. NeuroImage 19(3):1240–1249
Friston KJ, Penny W, Phillips C, Kiebel S, Hinton G, Ashburner J (2002) Classical and Bayesian inference in neuroimaging: theory. NeuroImage 16(2):465–483
Friston KJ, Harrison L, Penny W (2003) Dynamic causal modelling. NeuroImage 19(4):1273–1302
Gennatas ED et al (2017) Age-related effects and sex differences in gray matter density, volume, mass, and cortical thickness from childhood to young adulthood. J Neurosci 37(20):5065–5073
Goodfellow I, Bengio Y, Courville A (2016) Deep learning. MIT Press, Cambridge
Gustavsson A et al (2011) Cost of disorders of the brain in Europe 2010. Eur Neuropsychopharmacol 21(10):718–779
Hastie T, Tibshirani R (1990) Generalized additive models. Chapman & Hall, London
Insel TR, Cuthbert BN (2015) Medicine. Brain disorders? Precisely. Science 348(6234):499–500
James G et al (2013) An introduction to statistical learning: with applications in R. Springer, New York
Jebara T (2012) Machine learning: discriminative and generative. Springer Science & Business Media, Berlin
Jordan MI (2011) A message from the president: the era of big data. ISBA Bull 18(2):1–3
Jordan MI et al (1999) An introduction to variational methods for graphical models. Mach Learn 37(2):183–233
Mejia AF, Nebel MB, Shou H, Crainiceanu CM, Pekar JJ, Mostofsky S, Caffo B, Lindquist MA (2015) Improving reliability of subject-level resting-state fMRI parcellation with shrinkage estimators. NeuroImage 112:14–29
Miller RG (1981) Simultaneous statistical inference. Springer, Heidelberg
Miller KL et al (2016) Multimodal population brain imaging in the UK Biobank prospective epidemiological study. Nat Neurosci 19(11):1523–1536
Murphy KP (2012) Machine learning: a probabilistic perspective. MIT Press, Cambridge
Neyman J, Pearson ES (1933) On the problem of the most efficient tests of statistical hypotheses. Phil Trans R Soc Lond A Math Phys Sci 231:289–337
Smith SM, Nichols TE (2018) Statistical challenges in "big data" human neuroimaging. Neuron 97(2):263–268
Sudlow C et al (2015) UK Biobank: an open access resource for identifying the causes of a wide range of complex diseases of middle and old age. PLoS Med 12(3):e1001779
Takao H, Hayashi N, Ohtomo K (2013) Effects of the use of multiple scanners and of scanner upgrade in longitudinal voxel-based morphometry studies. J Magn Reson Imaging 38(5):1283–1291
Valiant LG (1984) A theory of the learnable. Commun ACM 27(11):1134–1142
Vapnik V (1998) Statistical learning theory. Wiley, New York
Varoquaux G, Gramfort A, Poline J-B, Thirion B (2010) Brain covariance selection: better individual functional connectivity models using population prior. Advances in neural information processing systems, pp 2334–2342
Wang H-T et al (2018) Dimensions of experience: exploring the heterogeneity of the wandering mind. Psychol Sci 29(1):56–71
Woo C-W et al (2017) Building better biomarkers: brain models in translational neuroimaging. Nat Neurosci 20(3):365–377
Yang Y, Wainwright MJ, Jordan MI (2016) On the computational complexity of high-dimensional Bayesian variable selection. Ann Stat 44(6):2497–2532

Phenomapping: Methods and Measures for Deconstructing Diagnosis in Psychiatry

7

Andre F. Marquand, Thomas Wolfers, and Richard Dinga

In most areas of medicine, the advent of biological tests to measure disease state has revolutionised diagnosis and treatment allocation. However, this is not the case in psychiatry, which is now virtually the last area of medicine where diseases are still diagnosed based on symptoms and biological tests to assist treatment allocation remain to be developed (Kapur et al. 2012). This is especially problematic because psychiatric disorders are all extremely heterogeneous, both in terms of their clinical presentation (which we refer to as 'clinical heterogeneity'), in terms of their underlying biological causes ('biological heterogeneity') and in terms of environmental factors ('environmental heterogeneity'). Even though diagnostic criteria have been periodically revised over the years, these sources of heterogeneity remain a substantial barrier to better understanding the causative mechanisms of psychiatric disorders and to developing optimal treatments. Indeed, there have been virtually no new therapeutic targets in psychiatry for decades.

A. F. Marquand
Donders Centre for Cognitive Neuroimaging, Donders Institute for Brain, Cognition and Behaviour, Radboud University, Nijmegen, The Netherlands

Department of Cognitive Neuroscience, Radboud University Medical Centre, Nijmegen, The Netherlands

Department of Neuroimaging, Centre for Neuroimaging Sciences, Institute of Psychiatry, King's College London, London, UK
e-mail: a.f.marquand@fcdonders.ru.nl

T. Wolfers
Donders Centre for Cognitive Neuroimaging, Donders Institute for Brain, Cognition and Behaviour, Radboud University, Nijmegen, The Netherlands

Department of Human Genetics, Radboud University Medical Centre, Nijmegen, The Netherlands

R. Dinga
Department of Psychiatry, Amsterdam Neuroscience and Amsterdam Public Health Research Institute, VU University Medical Center, Amsterdam, The Netherlands

I. C. Passos et al., *Personalized Psychiatry*,
https://doi.org/10.1007/978-3-030-03553-2_7

The overwhelmingly dominant paradigm in psychiatric research has been the case-control approach, which assumes that patient and control groups each form a distinct entity and completely ignores heterogeneity within cohorts. It has long been recognized that we must look beyond simple case-control comparisons to be able to deconstruct the heterogeneous phenotype of psychiatric disorders and, correspondingly, there have been many attempts to find data-driven reclassifications or stratifications of psychiatric disorders (Marquand et al. 2016b; Schnack 2018). The dominant approach has been to train unsupervised machine learning algorithms on the basis of symptoms or psychometric variables aiming to find data-driven subtypes of patients. Like the case-control approach, this assumes that patient cohorts can be cleanly partitioned into distinct subtypes. However, despite more than 40 years of effort, this approach has not converged upon a reproducible and clinically useful set of subtypes for any psychiatric disorder (Marquand et al. 2016b). Frustration with this lack of progress has led to several large-scale initiatives that aim to use many different biological and behavioural measures to finally bring the era of 'precision medicine' to psychiatry (Insel and Cuthbert 2015). The most prominent of these are the Research Domain Criteria (RDoC) initiative proposed by the National Institute of Mental Health in the USA (Insel et al. 2010) and the European Roadmap for Mental Health Research (ROAMER) (Schumann et al. 2014). The central feature of these initiatives is to move away from using only symptoms for disease classifications and instead to integrate biological and behavioural measures from different levels of analysis (e.g. genes, cells and circuits) and across different domains of functioning (e.g. positive affect, social processing). Although the short-term focus of RDoC and ROAMER is principally on research, the clear implication is that the current nosological classifications will eventually need to be revised. The way this is most popularly envisaged to occur is that by integrating across domains of functioning and across different biological and behavioural levels, psychiatric cohorts will be cleanly separable into subtypes that simultaneously cut across current diagnostic classifications and relate more closely to underlying brain systems (Insel and Cuthbert 2015). At the time of writing, it is eight years since RDoC was officially released, and it is fair to say that RDoC and similar initiatives have, to date, also provided only a modest yield. Whilst RDoC has driven substantial basic research,[1] there are still few successful attempts to stratify psychiatric disorders on the basis of biological systems and none that are close to challenging the current diagnostic criteria in clinical practice.

In view of the considerations above, in this chapter we will review the literature aiming to employ biological measures to stratify the phenotype of psychiatric disorders. First, we will briefly review the biological measures that useful for stratifying patient cohorts. Second, we give a brief conceptual overview of the different methodological approaches that have been employed for this purpose. Third, we will provide a focused review of studies that have used biological measures to derive stratification, in line with RDoC and ROAMER. Finally, we will

[1] See e.g. https://www.nimh.nih.gov/research-priorities/rdoc/nimh-rdoc-publications.shtml.

identify difficulties to finding reproducible and clinically meaningful stratifications and suggest new directions for the field. We will argue that a fixation on simple case-control type differences between well-defined subgroups has been a major limiting factor in finding reproducible and clinically meaningful stratifications.

7.1 Measuring Biology in Big Data Cohorts

In recent years clinical neuroscience has undergone a tectonic shift away from small, boutique studies towards big data cohorts. This entails an enormous increase both in the number of different measures of biology and behavior that are acquired and also in the size of the cohorts from which they are derived. For example, in genetics, large international consortia and data sharing initiatives have emerged that are providing increasing numbers of genome-wide significant hits for psychiatric disorders (e.g. Ripke et al. 2014). However, the effect size of all individual genetic variants discovered to date are small and even aggregation of many effects through polygenic risk scores only explains a tiny fraction of the variance in the phenotype of psychiatric disorders (e.g. Milaneschi et al. 2015). This means that genetic measures are probably better suited to profiling and validating prospective stratifications rather than deriving the stratifications themselves. At the same time, advances in brain imaging techniques now make it possible to measure many aspects of brain structure, function and connectivity non-invasively and in vivo. There are also now many large population-based studies that acquire a range of neuroimaging, behavioural and clinical measurements from large cohorts (e.g. the UK Biobank study (Miller et al. 2016) and the Human Connectome Project (Van Essen et al. 2013)). Together, this makes neuroimaging the most widely used—and arguably most promising—method for deriving biologically based stratifications of psychiatric disorders. However, many other measures also provide promising and potentially complimentary information for this purpose; for example, blood-based biomarkers (Lamers et al. 2013), continuous behavior monitoring from smartphones and wearable sensors (Torous et al. 2017) or electronic monitoring of continuous speech patterns (Bedi et al. 2015) but at the present time, these remain relatively unexplored for the purposes of stratification. Of course, different measures can also be combined via multi-modal data fusion (e.g. Wolfers et al. 2017), at the expense of increasing the complexity of the analytical pipeline. Consequently, the time has never been better for the application of machine learning based methods for data-driven stratification of psychiatric disorders on the basis of biological readouts. However, the advent of big data for clinical neuroscience brings particular analytical challenges. These include difficulties in scaling off-the-shelf approaches to high dimensional problems (Kriegel et al. 2009) and developing methods to capture clinically relevant variation across large cohorts of participants whilst separating that variation from nuisance variation (e.g. due to artefacts or site effects). Meaningful stratification of psychiatric disorders is therefore heavily dependent on the underlying analytical methodology.

7.2 Overview of Analytical Approaches for Stratification

The overwhelming majority of applications of machine learning methods to big data psychiatry have been *supervised* in the sense that they are provided with labels and the learning process consists of estimating a mapping between inputs (e.g. biomarkers) and outputs (e.g. diagnostic labels). There are many different approaches for supervised learning, including support vector machines (Boser et al. 1992), penalized linear models (Hastie et al. 2009) Bayesian approaches (Rasmussen and Williams 2006) and deep learning (LeCun et al. 2015). Whilst these differ with regard to the underlying model assumptions, associated estimation procedures and the accuracy with which they can predict the target labels, the fundamental idea behind all these approaches is the same in that the algorithm seeks to maximize the accuracy of predicting the label of new data points (Fig. 7.1a). In psychiatry, supervised learning has been widely used both for predicting diagnosis (Wolfers et al. 2015) and quantitative psychometric variables (e.g. Mwangi et al. 2012) on the basis of neuroimaging biomarkers.

The supervised approach is reasonable if the labels are known in advance and are both accurate and reliable. However, in psychiatry labelling errors are probably relatively common (e.g. due to clinical or biological heterogeneity in addition to misdiagnosis or comorbidity). With this in mind and since the aim of stratification is to understand variation within the disease group (i.e. independently from the diagnostic labels), supervised learning is not widely used for stratifying disease groups. One exception is supervised learning methods that include mechanisms for correcting errors in the labels (e.g. Young et al. 2013), which may be useful to identify atypical samples.

In contrast, in *unsupervised* learning, the machine learning algorithm is not provided with target values and learns to find structure in the data by applying heuristics encoded in each algorithm to the data. There are many types of unsupervised learning algorithm, including clustering, matrix factorization methods, latent variable models and anomaly detection methods (Hastie et al. 2009). Unsupervised learning approaches are often suitable for exploratory data analysis and are, on the face of it, well suited to stratifying the phenotype of psychiatric disorders and are widely used for this purpose (Marquand et al. 2016b; Schnack 2018).

7.3 Clustering

Clustering algorithms are probably the most widely used unsupervised approach in general and are certainly the most widely used methods for stratifying psychiatric disorders. The central idea is that an algorithm is trained to partition a set of data points (i.e. subjects) into different clusters on the basis of some measurements (e.g. derived from neuroimaging data), such that the samples in each cluster are more similar in some sense to one another than to those in the other clusters (Fig. 7.1b). This entails defining a measure of similarity or distance between data points (e.g.

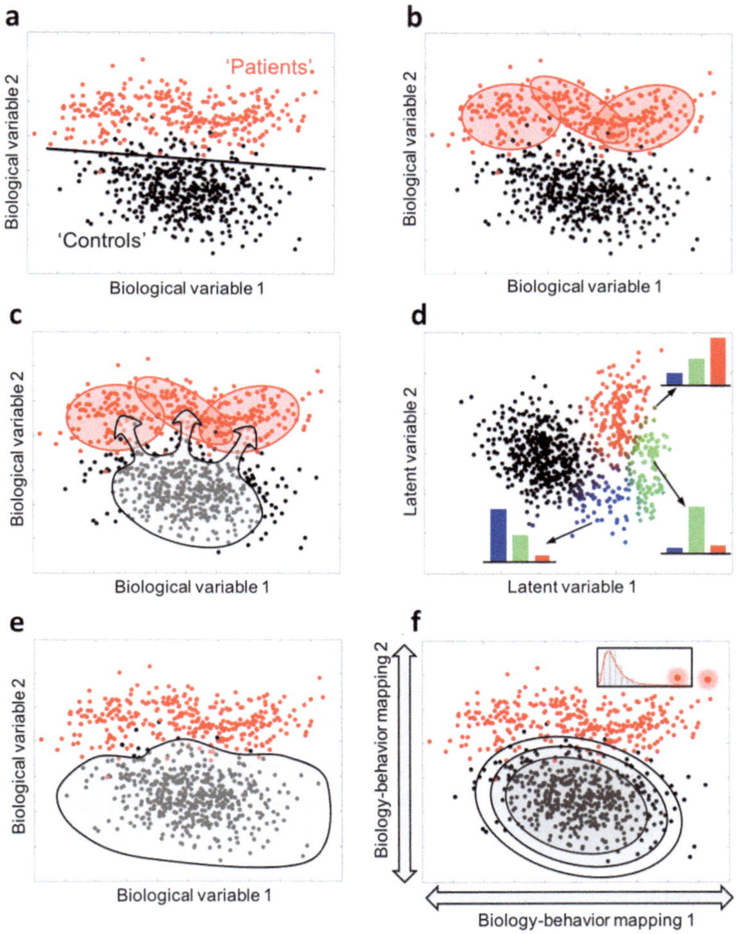

Fig. 7.1 Schematic overview of different approaches to parsing heterogeneity in psychiatric disorders on the basis of biological data. (**a**) Supervised learning approaches regard the patient and control groups as distinct entities, and thereby ignore heterogeneity within the data. (**b**) Clustering algorithms aim to partition one or both of the groups into discrete clusters. Here a Gaussian mixture model was estimated to partition the patient group into three clusters. Shown are the ellipsoids corresponding to one standard deviation from the cluster centers. (**c**) A hybrid method that combines clustering and distribution matching (Dong et al. 2016). Here the method estimates a set of three transformations that match the distribution of the control group to the distribution of the patient group. (**d**) A latent variable model that models symptoms as arising from a set of three latent disease processes (e.g. Zhang et al. 2016). The data are represented according to a set of latent variables (of which only two are shown as axes). Each datapoint from the patient group is colored according to the proportion of each latent process it expresses via red, blue or green hue. The loadings for three hypothetical data points are shown. (**e**) Outlier detection method that estimates a decision boundary enclosing the control group, aiming to detect patients as outliers (Mourao-Miranda et al. 2011). (**f**) Normative modelling approaches aim to estimate a normative distribution over a reference cohort such that the abnormality of each individual participant can be quantified via extreme value statistics. The extreme value abnormality score for one datapoint is shown in the inlay along with a fit extreme value distribution. Note that the normative distribution is defined with respect to a set of mappings between biology and behavior, analogous to 'growth charts' in somatic medicine (Marquand et al. 2016a). See text for further details

Euclidean distance or correlation) and the desired number of clusters. In the present work, we largely gloss over the differences between different clustering algorithms (e.g. K-means clustering, finite mixture modelling and graph-based clustering) and label these approaches simply as 'clustering'. We refer the interested reader to our previous work for more detail, where we provide a detailed introduction to some common clustering algorithms along with methodological considerations relating to their implementation (Marquand et al. 2016b).

7.4 Studies Subtyping Psychiatric Disorders on the Basis of Biology ('Biotyping')

As noted above, most applications to stratify psychiatric disorders on the basis of biology are based on the application of off-the-shelf clustering techniques, where the derived clusters are sometimes referred to as 'biotypes' (e.g. Clementz et al. 2016; Drysdale et al. 2017). One thing immediately apparent from a survey of the literature is a paucity of studies that report stratifications derived from biological measures, especially relative to the proliferation of applications of clustering algorithms to psychometric data (Marquand et al. 2016b). This is perhaps surprising given the strong motivation provided by the tight integration of research funding with initiatives such as RDoC and ROAMER (Insel et al. 2010; Schumann et al. 2014). One reason for this may be that biological data are often complex and high-dimensional with many different axes of variance. Clustering is a notoriously difficult problem in high dimensions (Kriegel et al. 2009) because many axes of variance may be artefactual or irrelevant and different axes may be important for different clusters within the same clustering solution. As a result, most applications reviewed here employ extreme dimensionality reduction, often training clustering algorithms on as few as two dimensions or alternatively use parameters from other models as features for clustering.

One of the earliest efforts to derive biotypes for stratifying psychiatric disorders was provided by Brodersen et al. (2014) who stratified a cohort of schizophrenia patients using Bayesian mixture model on the basis of parameters derived from a model of working memory estimated from functional magnetic resonance imaging (fMRI) data. This yielded three patient subgroups which differed in terms of symptom severity. Another study used structural connectivity measures derived from diffusion tensor imaging to stratify patients with first episode schizophrenia (Sun et al. 2015). This study reported two subtypes, which differed in terms of their profile of white matter abnormalities and symptom profile.

In a prominent study by Clementz et al. (2016), the authors derived a set of three biotypes from large cohort of patients with psychosis spectrum disorders using a broad panel of biomarkers, including neuropsychological, saccadic control and electroencephalography measures. These subtypes cut across classical diagnostic boundaries and had distinctive patterns of grey-matter reductions in a graded fashion such that one of the biotypes had patterns of reduction intermediate between the other two, a pattern also evident in relatives of the probands. Brain structural differences were further explored in a follow-up study (Ivleva et al. 2017), but since these analyses were performed on the same cohort, this cannot be considered a replication.

Another prominent study reported finding four biotypes of depression on the basis of mappings between resting state fMRI connectivity measures and symptoms derived from a multi-site cohort (Drysdale et al. 2017). These biotypes again crossed classical diagnostic boundaries and had differential characteristics with regard to symptoms and fMRI connectivity. The authors of this study performed limited validation of these subtypes on additional data samples and also demonstrated that the derived subtypes predicted treatment response (trans-cranial magnetic stimulation).

Finally, two studies from the same group have aimed to stratify attention-deficit hyperactivity disorder (ADHD) using functional connectivity measures derived from on fMRI (Gates et al. 2014; Costa Dias et al. 2015). These reported different numbers of clusters (3 and 5, respectively), and characterized the different subtypes in terms of their connectivity profiles although in the case of (Costa Dias et al. 2015), these were also related to symptom severity. As noted by the authors of these studies, this highlights that there are always multiple ways to partition cohorts using clustering algorithms, even based on the same data. These alternative solutions may be equally valid, for example when assessed according to different metrics (see below for further discussion).

7.5 Alternatives to Biotyping

There are multiple alternative analytical approaches for stratifying psychiatric disorders including hybrid methods that combine supervised learning with clustering (Varol et al. 2017), hybrid methods that combine distribution matching and clustering (Dong et al. 2016), methods that model the emergence of symptoms in individual subjects as deriving from a linear combination of latent disease factors (Ruiz et al. 2014; Zhang et al. 2016), outlier or anomaly detection methods (Mourao-Miranda et al. 2011) and normative modelling techniques that aim to chart variation in population cohorts and place each individual subject within the population range (Marquand et al. 2016a).

For example, the method proposed in (Dong et al. 2016) is a hybrid of clustering and distribution matching. This method was explicitly designed for structural brain imaging data and tackles heterogeneity within the patient cohort by training an algorithm that estimates a discrete set of transformations that warp the distribution of control participants to match the patient distribution (Fig. 7.1c). The intuition is that each of the different transformations encodes a different biotype. The method also provides a posterior probability measure quantifying the certainty with which each datapoint belongs to each biotype or, in other words, it provides a 'soft' clustering of the data. This was used to stratify a cohort of schizophrenia patients on the basis of structural MRI data (Honnorat et al. 2018), yielding three subtypes with different patterns of volumetric difference relative to control subjects.

Another alternative approach is based on the assumption that each individual expresses a set of latent disease factors to varying degrees, which together comprise an individualized symptom profile (Ruiz et al. 2014; Zhang et al. 2016). Such methods can be seen as relaxing the requirement that each subject belongs to a single cluster or subtype (Fig. 7.1d). A particularly promising approach along this line is topic modelling, which describes a collection of natural language processing techniques that aim to find a set of topics that occur frequently in a collection of documents such that each document is assumed to relate to multiple topics. For example, in (Zhang et al. 2016) the authors applied a common topic modelling technique—latent Dirichlet allocation (LDA; Blei et al. 2003)—to stratify Alzheimer's disease patients on the basis of structural MRI. In contrast to clustering approaches, LDA models disease in each individual patient (analogous to a 'document') as emerging from a pre-specified number of latent disease processes ('topics'), which are expressed to different degrees in different patients. Typically, LDA is framed as a probabilistic model, which can readily yield quantities of interest such as the probability that a given individual expresses a particular latent disease factor. In, the study by Zhang and colleagues (Zhang et al. 2016), the authors discovered three hierarchical latent disease factors characterized by different patterns of atrophy and different trajectories of cognitive decline.

In contrast, anomaly or outlier detection methods aim to estimate a predictive function or decision boundary that characterizes the support of the distribution of a healthy class. The intuition then is that 'abnormal' samples can be detected as outliers (Fig. 7.2e). Probably the most common approach in neuroimaging is the one-class support vector machine (OC-SVM; Sato et al. 2012). For example,

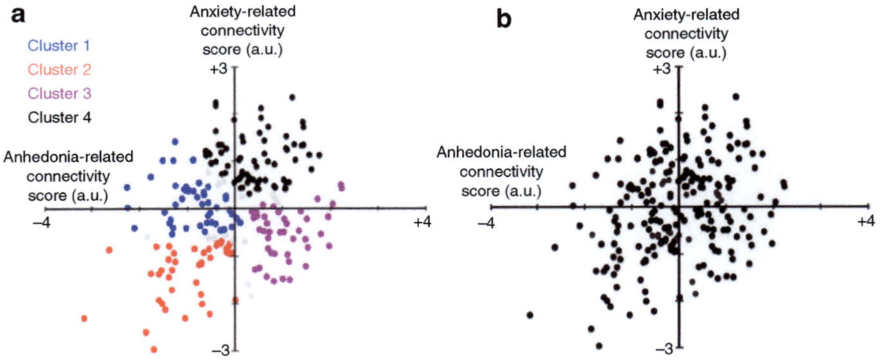

Fig. 7.2 Clustering algorithms can impose artificial categorical structure on underlying continuous variation. (**a**) Clustering solution from a study stratifying depression on the basis of symptoms and brain functional connectivity data (reproduced with permission from Drysdale et al. 2017). Each axis describes subject level loadings from canonical correlation analysis. Different colors represent different clusters and gray clusters are ambiguous data points that were excluded from the analysis when computing the distinctiveness of each cluster. (**b**) The same data with the cluster labels removed. It is clear that the evidence for clusters in the data is equivocal. The data could be equally well—and probably better—explained using a continuous model along two dimensions

Mourao-Miranda et al. (2011) applied this approach to fMRI data derived acquired while healthy participants and patients with depression were performing an affective processing task. The algorithm detected patients as outliers such that the degree of abnormality detected correlated with depression symptoms. The OC-SVM can be applied to relatively high dimensional problems, but only provides a decision boundary. In other words, it does not characterize the distribution statistically, nor provide estimates of variation within the distribution. For this, density estimation techniques (Hastie et al. 2009) could theoretically be applied, but these are largely limited to low dimensional problems.

Normative modelling (Marquand et al. 2016a; Fig. 7.2f) is an emerging statistical technique that approaches the stratification problem from a different perspective. Under this framework, a statistical model is estimated to chart centiles of variation in clinical cohorts such that each individual patient can be placed within the population distribution. This is analogous to the use of growth charts in somatic medicine to map child development (e.g. in terms of height or weight) as a function of age. At the heart of normative modelling is the estimation of mappings between psychometric variables and a quantitative biological readout that provide estimates of variation across the population. A straightforward example of such a mapping would be between chronological age and brain structure to form a 'brain growth chart', which is useful because most psychiatric disorders are rooted in an underlying trajectory of brain development (Insel 2014). However, the method is agnostic to the type of measures that are employed and it can be used to chart variation along any biological-behavioural axis. For example, in (Marquand et al. 2016a) a normative model of reward processing was estimated linking behavioural measures of delay discounting with reward-related brain activity. A second key ingredient in normative modelling is the use of extreme value statistics (Beirlant et al. 2004) to perform statistical inference over the aspects of the pattern that are most abnormal. The intuition behind this is that the method focusses on the most extreme differences from the expected pattern, following the notion that those differences are those most likely to be implicated in disease. In contrast, most of the more prevalent statistical techniques (e.g. t-statistics and analyses of variance) focus on central tendency, which is useful to detect mean differences between groups of participants but has limited ability to provide inferences about either individual participants, or about the aspects of the pattern that are most abnormal. The third key ingredient in normative modelling is the choice of the reference cohort. The most straightforward choice is to select only healthy participants such that deviations from the normative model can be interpreted as deviations from a healthy pattern. However, a different reference cohort could also be chosen, which includes subjects with different diagnoses as well as healthy subjects. If the prevalence of the different disorders within such a cohort matches the population prevalence, then such a cohort provides an accurate reflection of how abnormalities can be interpreted with respect to the population at large, which is often of interest in an epidemiological context.

Normative modelling has several distinguishing characteristics that set it apart from other methods. First, it provides statistical measures of deviation from a healthy pattern for each individual subject, in other words, providing personalized statistical predictions or 'fingerprints' that are at the heart of precision medicine (Insel and Cuthbert 2015; Kapur et al. 2012; Mirnezami et al. 2012). Second, normative modelling is completely agnostic to the diagnostic labels, which means they can be included as predictor variables to explain variance in the reference cohort. This is important because we must not overlook the discriminative power of diagnosis in many cases (Weinberger and Goldberg 2014). Third, normative modelling does not require that subjects share similar or overlapping patterns of abnormality and does not assume that the clinical cohort can be cleanly partitioned into subgroups although clustering algorithms can of course be trained on the deviations derived from normative models. This means it is useful to understand the variance structure in clinical cohorts where there are no clearly defined subtypes (e.g. where pathology may be better described as following a spectrum of functioning). In line with these considerations, some early application of normative modelling in schizophrenia, bipolar disorder, attention-deficit/hyperactivity disorder and autism spectrum disorders on the basis of structural MRI (Wolfers et al. 2018 https://www.ncbi.nlm.nih.gov/pubmed/30304337, https://www.biorxiv.org/content/early/2018/11/27/477596) are showing that group-level difference—or in other words differences in the 'average patient'—are only the 'tip of the iceberg'. Instead, most of the variation in psychiatric disorders is highly individualized and at the highest level of resolution (e.g. in terms of whole-brain voxel-level patterns of structural differences) does not provide compelling evidence for the existence of clusters.

7.6 Outlook and Challenges

There is a pervasive assumption that the optimal way to parse heterogeneity in psychiatric disorders is to partition the phenotype into subtypes. This assumption is effectively a recapitulation of the case-control approach and remains an implicit element of initiatives such as RDoC and ROAMER (Insel et al. 2010). Indeed, a criticism that has been leveled at RDoC is that it is in effect simply a new way to perform subtyping (Weinberger and Goldberg 2014). The subtyping approach has been successful in many other areas of medicine; for example, it has revolutionized oncology (Kalia 2015). However, we argue that it may not be optimal for psychiatric disorders. In psychiatry, few symptoms are unique to a single disorder and there are hundreds of genetic polymorphisms associated with most psychiatric disorders, all having small effect sizes and converging on similar symptoms (e.g. Betancur 2011; Ripke et al. 2014). Therefore, we argue that it may be unreasonable to expect cleanly separable subtypes for most disorders and alternative conceptual models may be more appropriate. One possibility is a 'watershed' model, which likens the pathophysiological process to a river system where many causative factors of small effect (e.g. genetic polymorphisms or environmental factors) begin as 'tributaries' and aggregate as they flow 'downstream' finding full expression in the syndromic expression of the disorder, akin to a river delta (Cannon 2016). Importantly, the watershed model does not necessarily imply that subtypes will be evident in the data.

We have reviewed elsewhere the extensive literature aiming to partition psychiatric disorders on the basis of symptoms and psychometric variables, where we noted that this approach has still not converged on a consistent set of subtypes despite considerable effort (Marquand et al. 2016b). Here, we have focused on attempts to find biological subtypes or biotypes of psychiatric disorders. Whilst the studies we have reviewed suggest that this may be possible, none of these have been completely replicated at the present time and the degree of external validation of the derived subtypes is modest. More importantly, it is important to recognize that all the biotyping studies we have reviewed employed clustering algorithms, which always yield a result. In other words, they will return a specified set of clusters, regardless of whether the data support clusters. In general, there is no universal metric to determine the 'optimal' number of clusters or to adjudicate between different clustering algorithms for a given dataset, and as a consequence a proliferation of various metrics have been proposed (Marquand et al. 2016b). Unlike supervised learning, where there is a clear measure of model quality (i.e. the accuracy with which new samples can be predicted), unsupervised learning models can be compared in many different ways (e.g. cluster separability, reproducibility or external validation accuracy) and it is usually not clear which is 'optimal'. Therefore, the final decision as to the 'best' clustering solution or algorithm often remains largely a matter of taste (Hastie et al. 2009). Moreover, most assessment metrics routinely used in practice are relative in the sense that they compare prospective clustering solutions with one another, but do not test the 'null' hypothesis that there are in fact clusters in the data. Various methods have been proposed that can be used to test whether clusters are 'really there' (Liu et al. 2008) and to compare the suitability of continuous, categorical and hybrid models for the data at hand (see Miettunen et al. 2016 for an overview). However, these approaches are currently underutilised for this purpose in psychiatry.

In line with this, it has been suggested that the biotypes reported by Clementz et al. (2016) may be better explained by a continuous dimensional representation relative to categorical subytpes (Barch 2017). We suggest here that the depression biotypes presented by Drysdale et al. (2017) may also reflect an imposed discretization of underlying continuous variation see Dinga et al. 2018 for further details https://www.biorxiv.org/content/early/2018/09/14/416321. In this study, biotypes were derived by training a clustering algorithm on two orthogonal mappings between brain connectivity and symptoms based on continuous subject loadings derived from canonical correlation analysis (Fig. 7.2a). Following cluster estimation, the authors increased the distinctiveness of their clusters by excluding ambiguous samples. Without this post-processing step, it becomes apparent that the evidence for the existence of clusters is equivocal in that the variation in the data could equally well be explained with two continuous axes (Fig. 7.2b). We emphasize that this does not imply that the findings reported are not biologically or clinically relevant, rather that the use of clustering algorithm imposes a categorical structure on the data that may not be optimal.

We reviewed several alternative methods to stratify psychiatric disorders. Whilst many of them are based on the same rationale as clustering approaches in that the phenotype can be split in to biotypes (Varol et al. 2017; Dong et al. 2016), these have features that ameliorate some of the problems inherent in applying 'off the shelf' algorithms to biometric data. For example, a common feature of many of these approaches (e.g. Marquand et al. 2016a; Varol et al. 2017; Dong et al. 2016) is that they break the symmetry inherent in the case-control and clustering approaches in the sense that they regard the disease cohort differently to the healthy cohort. This can be advantageous for stratifying psychiatric disorders because it allows the algorithm to focus on the manner in which patients deviate from a healthy pattern. It is especially beneficial in contexts where the clustering is performed on the basis of potentially high dimensional biological data because it means the clustering algorithm is less likely to detect nuisance variation that is of greater magnitude than disease-related effects (e.g. due to age or site).

Amongst the various methodological approaches we have reviewed, only a few methods are agnostic to the presence or absence of subtypes in the data (Miettunen et al. 2016; Marquand et al. 2016a; Mourao-Miranda et al. 2011; Zhang et al. 2016). Normative modeling is one promising example and whilst normative modelling can be used to derive features useful for clustering, its principal aim is to derive statistical estimates of deviation for each individual subject so that each subject can be compared to the normative or reference pattern. Another advantage of normative modelling is that it aims to estimate a supervised mapping and can therefore focus on the particular axes of variation (for example, the variation associated with a particular cognitive domain). Clearly, the development of alternative methods for stratifying the psychiatric phenotype are urgently needed.

As we briefly noted above, a major challenge for all methods is adequately and automatically dealing with artefacts in clinical datasets. There are many known sources of nuisance variance that are known to influence biological data and it is often the case that nuisance variation can be orders of magnitude greater than clinically relevant variation. This is particularly problematic because most stratification is performed in an unsupervised manner. A well-known example is head motion, which is widely acknowledged as a substantial challenge in fMRI studies (Van Dijk et al. 2012), and it is often the case that (in expectation) clinical groups move either more (e.g. ADHD) or less (e.g. depression) than healthy participants. These problems are compounded in large data cohorts, where data are often derived from multiple study sites, following different protocols. Moreover, nuisance variation often overlaps with clinically-relevant variation because important clinical or demographic variables are often not matched across study sites. Therefore finding techniques to deal with this optimally is a substantial ongoing challenge (Rao et al. 2017). One notable method that tackles this problem explicitly is the approach proposed by (Dong et al. 2016), which allows covariates such as age and sex to be specified so that the transformations estimated by the method take those into account.

7.7 Conclusions

In this chapter, we have reviewed literature aiming to use biological measures and big data cohorts to stratify psychiatric disorders. Whilst progress has clearly been made, there are major challenges for the field to overcome if we are to bring psychiatry closer towards precision medicine. We have argued that a widespread fixation on finding case-control type differences by partitioning the psychiatric phenotype into sharply defined clusters has impeded progress. Whilst successful in other areas of medicine, we argue that the complex multifactorial causes of psychiatric disorders combined with considerable overlap of symptoms across disorders mean that the biotyping approach may not be optimal in psychiatry. Currently only a few theoretical models have been proposed that do not assume the existence of clusters in the data (e.g. the 'watershed' model of Cannon 2016) and few analysis methods have been proposed that can fractionate psychiatric phenotypes without imposing clusters on the data. Alternative approaches are therefore urgently needed. Finally, we note that replication remains a major challenge for all methods. In line with the larger literature aiming to stratify psychiatric disorders (Marquand et al. 2016b; Schnack 2018), the studies reviewed here have—at best—performed a modicum of external validation, usually on the same cohort. At the time of writing, none of the studies we have reviewed in this chapter have been fully replicated to the degree that includes all steps in the analysis. This therefore remains an urgent priority.

References

Barch DM (2017) Biotypes: promise and pitfalls. Biol Psychiatry 82:2–3

Bedi G, Carillo F, Cecchi G, Sezak GF, Sigman M, Mota N, Ribeiro S, Javitt DC, Copelli M, Corcoran CM (2015) Automated analysis of free speech predicts psychosis onset in high-risk youths. Schizophrenia 1:15030

Beirlant J, Goegebeur Y, Teugels J, Segers J (2004) Statistics of extremes: theory and applications. Wiley, Sussex

Betancur C (2011) Etiological heterogeneity in autism spectrum disorders: more than 100 genetic and genomic disorders and still counting. Brain Res 1380:42–77

Blei DM, Ng AY, Jordan MI (2003) Latent Dirichlet allocation. J Mach Learn Res 3:993–1022

Boser B, Guyon I, Vapnik V (1992) A training algorithm for optimal margin classifiers. Proceedings of the fifth annual workshop on computational learning theory, vol 5, pp 144–152

Brodersen KH, Deserno L, Schlagenhauf F, Lin Z, Penny WD, Buhmann JM, Stephan KE (2014) Dissecting psychiatric spectrum disorders by generative embedding. Neuroimage Clin 4:98–111

Cannon TD (2016) Deciphering the genetic complexity of schizophrenia. JAMA Psychiat 73:5–6

Clementz BA, Sweeney JA, Hamm JP, Ivleva EI, Ethridge LE, Pearlson GD, Keshavan MS, Tamminga CA (2016) Identification of distinct psychosis biotypes using brain-based biomarkers. Am J Psychiatry 173:373–384

Costa Dias TG, Iyer SP, Carpenter SD, Cary RP, Wilson VB, Mitchell SH, Nigg JT, Fair DA (2015) Characterizing heterogeneity in children with and without ADHD based on reward system connectivity. Dev Cogn Neurosci 11:155–174

Dong AY, Honnorat N, Gaonkar B, Davatzikos C (2016) CHIMERA: clustering of heterogeneous disease effects via distribution matching of imaging patterns. IEEE Trans Med Imaging 35:612–621

Drysdale AT, Grosenick L, Downar J, Dunlop K, Mansouri F, Meng Y, Fetcho RN, Zebley B, Oathes DJ, Etkin A, Schatzberg AF, Sudheimer K, Keller J, Mayberg HS, Gunning FM, Alexopoulos GS, Fox MD, Pascual-Leone A, Voss HU, Casey BJ, Dubin MJ, Liston C (2017) Resting-state connectivity biomarkers define neurophysiological subtypes of depression. Nat Med 23:28–38

Gates KM, Molenaar PCM, Iyer SP, Nigg JT, Fair DA (2014) Organizing heterogeneous samples using community detection of GIMME-derived resting state functional networks. PLoS One 9(3):e91322

Hastie T, Tibshirani R, Friedman J (2009) The elements of statistical learning. Springer, New York

Honnorat J, Dong A, Meizenzahl-Lechner E, Koutsoleris N, Davatzikos C (2018) Neuroanatomical heterogeneity of schizophrenia revealed by semi-supervised machine learning methods. In press

Insel TR (2014) Mental disorders in childhood shifting the focus from behavioral symptoms to neurodevelopmental trajectories. JAMA 311:1727–1728

Insel TR, Cuthbert BN (2015) Brain disorders? Precisely. Science 348:499–500

Insel T, Cuthbert B, Garvey M, Heinssen R, Pine DS, Quinn K, Sanislow C, Wang P (2010) Research domain criteria (RDoC): toward a new classification framework for research on mental disorders. Am J Psychiatry 167:748–751

Ivleva EI, Clementz BA, Dutcher AM, Arnold SJM, Jeon-Slaughter H, Aslan S, Witte B, Poudyal G, Lu H, Meda SA, Pearlson GD, Sweeney JA, Keshavan MS, Tamminga CA (2017) Brain structure biomarkers in the psychosis biotypes: findings from the bipolar-schizophrenia network for intermediate phenotypes. Biol Psychiatry 82:26–39

Kalia M (2015) Biomarkers for personalized oncology: recent advances and future challenges. Metabolism 64:S16–S21

Kapur S, Phillips AG, Insel TR (2012) Why has it taken so long for biological psychiatry to develop clinical tests and what to do about it? Mol Psychiatry 17:1174–1179

Kriegel H-P, Kroeger P, Zimek A (2009) Clustering high-dimensional data: a survey on subspace clustering, pattern-based clustering, and correlation clustering. ACM Trans Knowl Discov Data 3:1–58

Lamers F, Vogelzangs N, Merikangas KR, De Jonge P, Beekman ATF, Penninx BWJH (2013) Evidence for a differential role of HPA-axis function, inflammation and metabolic syndrome in melancholic versus atypical depression. Mol Psychiatry 18:692–699

Lecun Y, Bengio Y, Hinton G (2015) Deep learning. Nature 521:436–444

Liu Y, Hayes DN, Nobel A, Marron JS (2008) Statistical significance of clustering for high-dimension, low-sample size data. J Am Stat Assoc 103:1281–1293

Marquand AF, Rezek I, Buitelaar J, Beckmann CF (2016a) Understanding heterogeneity in clinical cohorts using normative models: beyond case-control studies. Biol Psychiatry 80:552–561

Marquand AF, Wolfers T, Mennes M, Buitelaar J, Beckmann CF (2016b) Beyond lumping and splitting: a review of computational approaches for stratifying psychiatric disorders. Biol Psychiatry Cogn Neurosci Neuroimaging 1:433–447

Miettunen J, Nordstrom T, Kaakinen M, Ahmed AO (2016) Latent variable mixture modeling in psychiatric research—a review and application. Psychol Med 46:457–467

Milaneschi Y, Lamers F, Peyrot WJ, Abdellaoui A, Willemsen G, Hottenga J-J, Jansen R, Mbarek H, Dehghan A, Lu C, CHARGE Inflammation Working Group, Boomsma DI, Penninx BWHJ (2015) Polygenic dissection of major depression clinical heterogeneity. In press

Miller KL, Alfaro-Almagro F, Bangerter NK, Thomas DL, Yacoub E, Xu JQ, Bartsch AJ, Jbabdi S, Sotiropoulos SN, Andersson JLR, Griffanti L, Douaud G, Okell TW, Weale P, Dragonu J, Garratt S, Hudson S, Collins R, Jenkinson M, Matthews PM, Smith SM (2016) Multimodal population brain imaging in the UK Biobank prospective epidemiological study. Nat Neurosci 19:1523–1536

Mirnezami R, Nicholson J, Darzi A (2012) Preparing for precision medicine. N Engl J Med 366:489–491

Mourao-Miranda J, Hardoon DR, Hahn T, Marquand AF, Williams SCR, Shawe-Taylor J, Brammer M (2011) Patient classification as an outlier detection problem: an application of the one-class support vector machine. Neuroimage 58:793–804

Mwangi B, Matthews K, Steele JD (2012) Prediction of illness severity in patients with major depression using structural MR brain scans. J Magn Reson Imaging 35:64–71

Rao A, Monteiro JM, Mourao-Miranda J, Alzheimers Dis I (2017) Predictive modelling using neuroimaging data in the presence of confounds. Neuroimage 150:23–49

Rasmussen CE, Williams C (2006) Gaussian processes for machine learning. MIT Press, Cambridge

Ripke S, Neale BM, Corvin A, Walters JTR, Farh K-H, Holmans PA, Lee P, Bulik-Sullivan B, Collier DA, Huang H, Pers TH, Agartz I, Agerbo E, Albus M, Alexander M, Amin F, Bacanu SA, Begemann M, Belliveau RA Jr, Bene J, Bergen SE, Bevilacqua E, Bigdeli TB, Black DW, Bruggeman R, Buccola NG, Buckner RL, Byerley W, Cahn W, Cai G, Campion D, Cantor RM, Carr VJ, Carrera N, Catts SV, Chambert KD, Chan RCK, Chen RYL, Chen EYH, Cheng W, Cheung EFC, Chong SA, Cloninger CR, Cohen D, Cohen N, Cormican P, Craddock N, Crowley JJ, Curtis D, Davidson M, Davis KL, Degenhardt F, Del Favero J, Demontis D, Dikeos D, Dinan T, Djurovic S, Donohoe G, Drapeau E, Duan J, Dudbridge F, Durmishi N, Eichhammer P, Eriksson J, Escott-Price V, Essioux L, Fanous AH, Farrell MS, Frank J, Franke L, Freedman R, Freimer NB, Friedl M, Friedman JI, Fromer M, Genovese G, Georgieva L, Giegling I, Giusti-Rodriguez P, Godard S, Goldstein JI, Golimbet V, Gopal S, Gratten J, De Haan L, Hammer C, Hamshere ML, Hansen M, Hansen T, Haroutunian V, Hartmann AM, Henskens FA, Herms S, Hirschhorn JN, Hoffmann P, Hofman A, Hollegaard MV, Hougaard DM, Ikeda M, Joa I et al (2014) Biological insights from 108 schizophrenia-associated genetic loci. Nature 511:421–427

Ruiz FJR, Valera I, Blanco C, Perez-Cruz F (2014) Bayesian nonparametric comorbidity analysis of psychiatric disorders. J Mach Learn Res 15:1215–1247

Sato JR, Rondina JM, Mourao-Miranda J (2012) Measuring abnormal brains: building normative rules in neuroimaging using one-class support vector machines. Front Neurosci 6:178

Schnack H (2018) Improving individual predictions: machine learning approaches for detecting and attacking heterogeneity in schizophrenia (and other psychiatric disorders). Schizophr Res. In press

Schumann G, Binder EB, Holte A, De Kloet ER, Oedegaard KJ, Robbins TW, Walker-Tilley TR, Bitter I, Brown VJ, Buitelaar J, Ciccocioppo R, Cools R, Escera C, Fleischhacker W, Flor H, Frith CD, Heinz A, Johnsen E, Kirschbaum C, Klingberg T, Lesch K-P, Lewis S, Maier W, Mann K, Martinot J-L, Meyer-Lindenberg A, Mueller CP, Mueller WE, Nutt DJ, Persico A, Perugi G, Pessiglione M, Preuss UW, Roiser JP, Rossini PM, Rybakowski JK, Sandi C, Stephan KE, Undurraga J, Vieta E, Van Der Wee N, Wykes T, Maria Haro J, Wittchen HU (2014) Stratified medicine for mental disorders. Eur Neuropsychopharmacol 24:5–50

Sun H, Lui S, Yao L, Deng W, Xiao Y, Zhang W, Huang X, Hu J, Bi F, Li T, Sweeney JA, Gong Q (2015) Two patterns of white matter abnormalities in medication-naive patients with first-episode schizophrenia revealed by diffusion tensor imaging and cluster analysis. JAMA Psychiat 72:678–686

Torous J, Onnela JP, Keshavan M (2017) New dimensions and new tools to realize the potential of RDoC: digital phenotyping via smartphones and connected devices. Transl Psychiatry 7(3):e1053

Van Dijk KRA, Sabuncu MR, Buckner RL (2012) The influence of head motion on intrinsic functional connectivity MRI. Neuroimage 59:431–438

Van Essen DC, Smith SM, Barch DM, Behrens TEJ, Yacoub E, Ugurbil K, Consortium WU-MH (2013) The WU-minn human connectome project: an overview. Neuroimage 80:62–79

Varol E, Sotiras A, Davatzikos C, Alzheimer's Disease Neuroimaging Initiative (2017) HYDRA: revealing heterogeneity of imaging and genetic patterns through a multiple max-margin discriminative analysis framework. Neuroimage 145:346–364

Weinberger DR, Goldberg TE (2014) RDoCs redux. World Psychiatry 13:36–38

Wolfers T, Buitelaar JK, Beckmann C, Franke B, Marquand AF (2015) From estimating activation locality to predicting disorder: a review of pattern recognition for neuroimaging-based psychiatric diagnostics. Neurosci Biobehav Rev. In press

Wolfers T, Arenas AL, Onnink AMH, Dammers J, Hoogman M, Zwiers MP, Buitelaar JK, Franke B, Marquand AF, Beckmann CF (2017) Refinement by integration: aggregated effects of multimodal imaging markers on adult ADHD. J Psychiatry Neurosci 42:386–394

Young J, Ashburner J, Ourselin S (2013) Wrapper methods to correct mislabelled training data. 3rd international workshop on pattern recognition in neuroimaging. IEEE, Philadelphia

Zhang XM, Mormino EC, Sun NB, Sperling RA, Sabuncu MR, Yeo BT, Alzheimer's Disease Neuroimaging Initiative (2016) Bayesian model reveals latent atrophy factors with dissociable cognitive trajectories in Alzheimer's disease. Proc Natl Acad Sci U S A 113:E6535–E6544

8 How to Integrate Data from Multiple Biological Layers in Mental Health?

Rogers F. Silva and Sergey M. Plis

8.1 Overview

The human brain is a massively parallel learning machine that contains multiple highly complex structurally and functionally overlapping subsystems, with processes occurring at different temporal and spatial scales, and interacting with every other bodily system through the peripheral nervous system. In order to gain a more complete understanding of its organization and function, information from various layers of this complex set of biological processes must be evaluated *simultaneously*, in a truly synergistic fashion.

To begin with, collecting such information *directly* often entails invasive procedures that are restricted to very narrow patient populations, such as with electrocorticography (ECoG) and deep brain electrodes. However, in order to be also able to study much broader healthy population baselines, it is necessary to pursue less invasive routes. Specifically, those enabled by means of indirect measurements from secondary biological processes such as cerebral blood flow and induced electromagnetic fields. While noninvasiveness often comes at the cost of blurring some of the true underlying neurological signals, the greater availability of subjects enables normative as well as comparative analyses, with far greater statistical power due to the substantially increased sample sizes. Furthermore, one must also be mindful of inherent sensor and device limitations dictating the temporal and spatial resolutions of the data, which ultimately yield only fragments of the measured processes, adding yet another layer of complexity to the data.

With these in mind, it is sensible to hereon broadly associate the term *biological layer* with different *imaging modalities*, i.e., the signal of some direct or indirect neurobiological process captured by a device. Common examples of

R. F. Silva · S. M. Plis (✉)
The Mind Research Network, Albuquerque, NM, USA
e-mail: splis@mrn.org

I. C. Passos et al., *Personalized Psychiatry*,
https://doi.org/10.1007/978-3-030-03553-2_8

such modalities include, but are not limited to, structural, functional, and diffusion weighted/spectrum magnetic resonance imaging (sMRI, fMRI, and DWI/DSI, respectively), electro- and magneto-encephalography (E/MEG), functional near-infrared spectroscopy (fNIRS), x-rays, computerized tomography (CT), positron emission tomography (PET), single-photon emission CT (SPECT), intracranial electrodes, genetic material information such as DNA microarrays, single nucleotide polymorphism and DNA methylation, as well as metabolomic and microbiome derivatives, etc. Demographic and behavioral information on individuals and populations of interest are also going to be considered modalities for the purposes of this chapter.

Under this broad definition, we will focus on the integration of biological layers by means of *direct joint analysis of all modalities* available. Joint analyses are those which simultaneously utilize data from all modalities in a synergistic way and, thus, can be categorized as *data fusion* approaches. A key requirement for these kinds of analyses is that the information contained in each modality have been collected *on the same subject* so that the data are naturally linked. For the same reason, whenever feasible, simultaneous measurements are also preferred over (and likely more informative than) measures from different sessions since that entails a stronger link between modalities.

The goal of integrating multiple biological layers is to identify the neurobiological processes underlying the measurements recorded in the data in order to understand their function, structure, and interaction. Ideally, we want to make predictions about these processes and be able to explain their causal mechanisms. Each biological layer is itself only a part of the underlying process. For example, blood flow picked up by fMRI and electrical activity of neurons registered by EEG are parts of the same process of neural activity. Only together—plus many other additional pieces of information, such as neural connectivity routes—they provide a complete picture of the underlying mechanism. Available *imaging modalities* provide a (partial) glimpse on many of the individual processes within a functioning brain. When any of them are used, we are dealing not only with the partial nature of the biological layers but also with the fact that each of the layers is measured with uncertainty that is different for each imaging modality. Fortunately, the uncertainty introduced by the employed imaging modality is often different for each biological layer and, optimistically, can cancel if the imaging modalities are properly combined. The difference in uncertainties is illustrated by MEG and fMRI, where the former has arguably greater spatial, while the latter has greater temporal uncertainty relative to the underlying process of neural activity. Given the insufficient nature of each modality, the only way we can build a complete understanding of the brain is by combining these complementary sources. Together, the limited views from each modality allow us to peer into the underlying biostructure. In summary, scientific discovery with data fusion should proceed in cycles: measuring different physical processes at various biological and temporal scales, synthesizing that information using specific methods, understanding the underlying processes identified, and repeating with the gained insights.

In the following sections, we will discuss two principled approaches to fusion of multimodal imaging data. The first is blind source separation (BSS), which deals directly with the problem of identifying underlying sources utilizing statistical (un)correlation and (in)dependence within and across modalities. The second is deep learning, focusing on multimodal architectures for classification, embedding, and segmentation.

8.2 Blind Source Separation Methods

Blind source separation (BSS) deals with the general problem of *blindly* recovering hidden source signals $\mathbf{y}$ from a dataset $\mathbf{x}$, i.e., without any knowledge of the function $\mathbf{f}$ nor the parameters $\boldsymbol{\theta}$ which generate $\mathbf{x} = \mathbf{f}(\mathbf{y}, \boldsymbol{\theta})$. It can be organized into subproblems according to the number of datasets contained in $\mathbf{x}$ and the presence of subsets of $\mathbf{y}$ grouped as multidimensional sources within any single dataset. The following taxonomy arranges BSS subproblems by increasing complexity:

SDU In the single-dataset unidimensional (SDU) subproblem, $\mathbf{x}$ consists of a single dataset whose sources are *not* grouped. This is the seminal and most studied area of BSS, including classical problems such as independent component analysis (ICA) (Comon 1994; Bell and Sejnowski 1995; Hyvärinen and Erkki 1997) and second-order blind identification (SOBI) (Belouchrani et al. 1993; Yeredor 2000).

MDU In the multidataset unidimensional (MDU) subproblem, $\mathbf{x}$ consists of one or more datasets and, while *no* sources are grouped within any dataset, multidimensional sources containing *a single source from each dataset* may occur. Examples in this area include canonical correlation analysis (CCA) (Hotelling 1936), partial least squares (PLS) (Wold 1966), and independent vector analysis (IVA) (Adalı et al. 2014; Kim et al. 2006).

SDM In the single-dataset multidimensional (SDM) subproblem, $\mathbf{x}$ consists of a single dataset with one or more multidimensional sources. Examples include multidimensional ICA (MICA) (Cardoso 1998; Lahat et al. 2012) and independent subspace analysis (ISA) (Hyvärinen and Köster 2006; Szabó et al. 2012).

MDM In the general multidataset multidimensional (MDM) problem, $\mathbf{x}$ contains one or more datasets, each with one or more multidimensional sources that may group further with single or multidimensional sources from the remaining datasets. Examples include multidataset ISA (MISA) (Silva et al. 2014a,b) and joint ISA (JISA) (Lahat and Jutten 2015).

These definitions support a natural hierarchy in which subproblems are contained within one another, with SDU problems being a special case of MDU, SDM, and MDM problems, and MDU and SDM problems being special cases of MDM.

The "blind" property of BSS makes it particularly powerful and attractive in the absence of a precise model of the measured system and with data confounded by noise of unknown or variable characteristics. These are marked signatures of multimodal fusion applications exploring the extreme complexities of the human brain, with largely heterogeneous noise characteristics and artifacts occurring across data types. This is a clear indicator that BSS is ripe for application in multimodal fusion of human brain data, as we will illustrate in the following sections. To begin with, we present the mathematical notation for the general MDM problem, followed by an example of an application of ICA to fusion of brain MRI and EEG features. We then briefly review other more advanced applications of BSS to multimodal fusion of brain imaging data before moving on to deep learning methods.

8.2.1 General MDM Problem Statement

Given N observations of $M \geq 1$ datasets (or modalities), identify an unobservable latent source random vector (r.v.) $\mathbf{y} = \left[\mathbf{y}_1^T \cdots \mathbf{y}_M^T\right]^T$, $\mathbf{y}_m = [y_1 \cdots y_{C_m}]^T$, that relates to the observed r.v. $\mathbf{x} = \left[\mathbf{x}_1^T \cdots \mathbf{x}_M^T\right]^T$, $\mathbf{x}_m = [x_1 \cdots x_{V_m}]^T$, via a mixture function $\mathbf{f}(\mathbf{y}, \boldsymbol{\theta})$, where $\boldsymbol{\theta}$ are the function parameters. Both $\mathbf{y}$ and the transformation represented by $\mathbf{f}(\mathbf{y}, \boldsymbol{\theta})$ have to be learned blindly, i.e., without explicit knowledge of either of them. In order to make this problem tractable, a few assumptions are required:

1. the number of latent sources C_m in each dataset is known by the experimenter;
2. $\mathbf{f}(\mathbf{y}, \boldsymbol{\theta}) = \mathbf{A}\mathbf{y}$, i.e., a *linear* transformation, with $\boldsymbol{\theta} = \mathbf{A}$;
3. $\mathbf{A}$ is a $\bar{V} \times \bar{C}$ block diagonal matrix with M blocks, representing a separable layout structure such that $\mathbf{x}_m = \mathbf{A}_m \mathbf{y}_m$, $m = 1 \ldots M$, where $\bar{C} = \sum_{m=1}^{M} C_m$, $\bar{V} = \sum_{m=1}^{M} V_m$, and each block $\mathbf{A}_m$ is $V_m \times C_m$;
4. some of the latent sources in $\mathbf{y}$ are statistically related to each other and this *dependence* is undirected (non-causal), occurring both within or across datasets;
5. related sources establish subspaces (or source *groups*) $\mathbf{y}_k$, $k = 1 \ldots K$, with both K and the specific subspace compositions known by the experimenter and prescribed in an assignment matrix $\mathbf{P}_k$.

Under these assumptions, recovering the sources $\mathbf{y}$ amounts to finding a linear transformation $\mathbf{W}$ of the observed datasets via the unmixing function $\mathbf{y} = \mathbf{W}\mathbf{x}$. This is accurate when $\mathbf{W} = \mathbf{A}^{-}$, the pseudo-inverse of $\mathbf{A}$, which implies $\mathbf{W}$ is also block diagonal, thus satisfying $\mathbf{y}_m = \mathbf{W}_m \mathbf{x}_m$. Source subspaces are then estimated as $\mathbf{y}_k = \mathbf{P}_k \mathbf{W}\mathbf{x}$. In the following, unless noted otherwise, the m-th $V_m \times N$ data matrix is denoted as $\mathbf{X}_m$, containing N observations of $\mathbf{x}_m$ along its columns; $\mathbf{X}$ denotes a $\bar{V} \times N$ matrix concatenating all $\mathbf{X}_m$. Figure 8.1 illustrates this model, starting with its special cases.

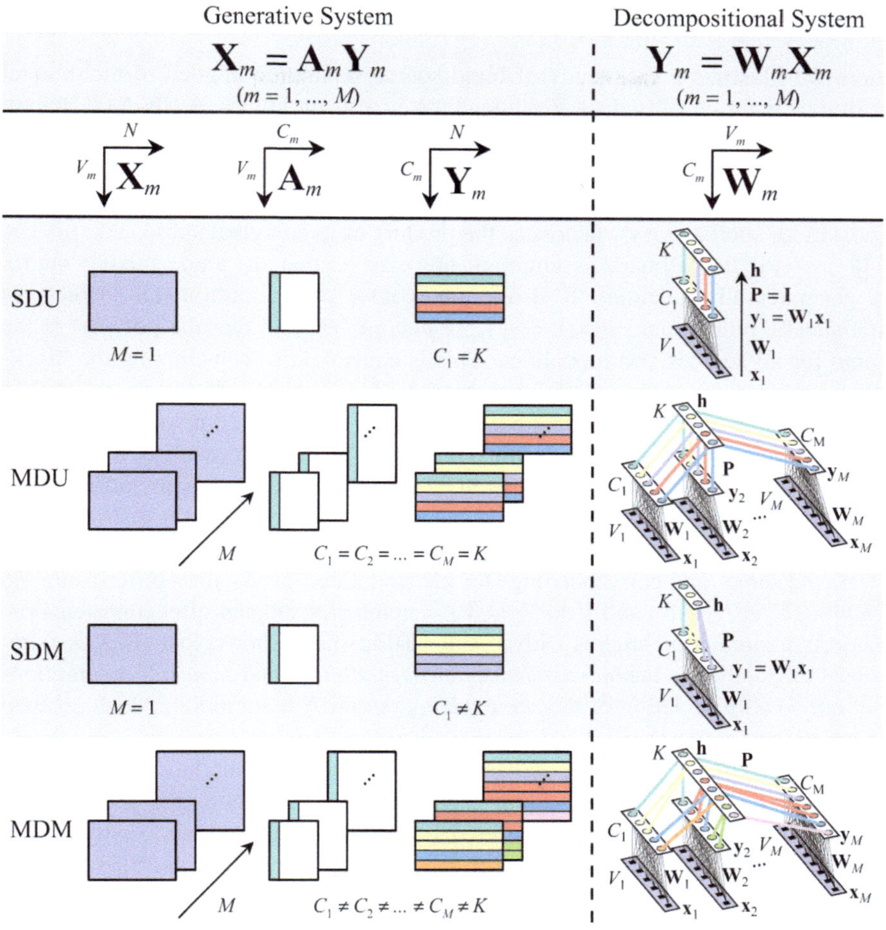

Fig. 8.1 Side-by-side illustration of the generative and decompositional system representations of linear BSS problems. Each of M datasets (or modalities) is represented by a matrix $\mathbf{X}_m$, with the same number of observations N along the columns. A column of $\mathbf{X}_m$ is represented by $\mathbf{x}_m$ (likewise for $\mathbf{Y}_m$ and $\mathbf{y}_m$). The generative system representation describes how each modality is generated from a set of underlying sources, in this case by a linear transformation of the source matrix $\mathbf{Y}_m$ through $\mathbf{A}_m$, the *mixing* matrix. In the general case, both $\mathbf{A}_m$ and $\mathbf{Y}_m$ are unique to each modality. Associations across modalities are represented by subspaces (K), which are collections of statistically *dependent* sources. *This dependence is indicated by coloring sources with the same color*. The linearity of the generative system implies linearity of the decompositional system. The decompositional representation indicates how source estimation occurs, namely by decomposing modalities into their underlying sources via a linear transformation of each modality $\mathbf{X}_m$ through $\mathbf{W}_m$, the *unmixing* matrix. In this representation, each V_m-dimensional column $\mathbf{x}_m$ is linearly transformed into a C_m-dimensional vector $\mathbf{y}_m$, whose elements (the individual sources) are then composed with other sources into subspaces, according to an *assignment* matrix $\mathbf{P}$ and non-linearity $\mathbf{h}(\cdot)$ ensuing from the choice of activation and objective functions

8.2.2 Case Study: Multimodal Fusion with Joint ICA

Here we illustrate a case study of blind source separation applied to multimodal fusion of brain imaging data. Specifically, we focus on joint ICA (jICA) (Calhoun and Adalı 2009), a very attractive model because of its simplicity as an MDU-type model cleverly designed to operate like an SDU-type model. Like ICA, it seeks statistically independent $\mathbf{y}_k$ such that the joint probability density function (pdf) of all sources, $p(\mathbf{y})$, factors as the product of its marginal subspaces: $p(\mathbf{y}) = \prod_{k=1}^{K} p(\mathbf{y}_k)$. Its hallmark assumption, however, is that the same mixing matrix $\mathbf{A}$ generates all modalities. It also assumes *none* of the multimodal sources are statistically related, i.e., $p(\mathbf{y}_k) = \prod_{m=1}^{M} p(y_{mk})$, $\forall k$, and that the pdf $p(\cdot)$ is the same for all sources and modalities. This is equivalent to constraining the block-diagonal structure in the MDU subproblem to $\mathbf{A}_m = \mathbf{A}$, $\forall m$. However, rather than choosing an M-dimensional joint pdf for $\mathbf{y}_k$, jICA combines corresponding sources y_{mk} of $\mathbf{y}_k$ into a single one-dimensional pdf $p(y_i)$, where i is the source number and $i = k$, which conveniently permits an SDU-type solution utilizing any off-the-shelf ICA algorithm after simple side-by-side concatenation of the data matrices from each modality. This also eliminates the requirement that the number of observations N be the same (and corresponding) for all modalities, so N_1 may differ from N_2, yielding $N = N_1 + N_2$ and $V = V_1 = V_2 =$ number of subjects after concatenation. Thorough simulation studies (Silva et al. 2014c) have shown that jICA is fairly robust to violation of the *independence across modalities* and *same pdf* assumptions but *not* so with violation of the *same mixing matrix* $\mathbf{A}$ assumption, which resulted in poorer performance.

Three seminal works have utilized joint ICA for multimodal fusion in brain imaging as a means to draw upon each modality's strengths and provide new information about the brain not offered by either modality alone. Firstly, fusion of multitask fMRI features (Calhoun et al. 2006b) promoted the direct use of data modeled at the subject level in a "unified analytic framework" for joint examination of multitask fMRI activations, leading to interesting, new findings that were missed by traditional analyses. Blood oxygen level dependent (BOLD) fMRI scans from 15 healthy control subjects and 15 outpatients with chronic schizophrenia matched for age, gender, and task difficulty were collected during two separate tasks: an auditory "oddball" task (AOD) and a Sternberg working memory task (SB). For every subject, regressors were created by modeling correct responses to task-specific stimuli as delta functions convolved with a canonical hemodynamic response function (HRF). These regressors plus their temporal derivatives and an intercept were included in a general linear model (GLM) of multiple regression fit to every voxel timeseries. The resulting AOD target-versus-standard contrast and SB recognition (or recall) contrast against baseline from each subject (averaged over all levels of difficulty) were corrected for amplitude bias due to spatially varying latencies using derivative boost and then arranged into matrices $\mathbf{X}_1$ and $\mathbf{X}_2$ (AOD and SB features, respectively). Both matrices were normalized to have the same average sum-of-squares before concatenation, followed by (joint) PCA data reduction and ICA, using the extended Infomax algorithm to adaptively allow some flexibility on the combined source pdfs $p(y_i)$ and, thus, mitigate potential side effects of violations to the same pdf assumption. Finally, rather than testing thousands of voxels, two-sample t-tests on each column of the shared subject expression profiles $\mathbf{A}$ were conducted to identify sources with significant group differences in coupling (regarded as a relative measure of the degree of group-level functional connectivity difference). For the identified source (Fig. 8.2), the joint probability of the multitask *data* $p(x_1(n_1), x_2(n_2))$ was assessed by means of subject-specific joint histograms, where n_m were the voxel indexes for modality m sorted from largest to smallest by their *source* values y_{mn} over all $n = 1, \ldots, N$, on voxels surviving an arbitrary $|Z| > 3.5$ threshold.

Secondly, fusion of fMRI and sMRI features (Calhoun et al. 2006a) enabled a direct study of the interactions and associations between changes in fMRI activation and changes in brain structure contained in sMRI data. Utilizing probabilistic segmentation (soft classification) maps of gray matter (GM) concentration derived from T_1-weighted sMRI images and the AOD target-versus-standard contrast from the same subjects described above, feature matrices $\mathbf{X}_1$ and $\mathbf{X}_2$ were created, respectively. The sign of alternating voxels was flipped in GM maps to yield zero-mean maps for each subject (this step was undone after jICA estimation and before histogram computation and visualizations). Before concatenation of $\mathbf{X}_1$ and $\mathbf{X}_2$, both matrices were normalized to have the same average sum-of-squares. Joint PCA data reduction and ICA followed, using the extended Infomax algorithm to adaptively allow some flexibility on the combined source pdfs $p(y_i)$ and, thus, mitigate potential side effects of violations to the same pdf assumption. Like in the multitask case, two-sample t-tests on each column of the shared subject expression profiles $\mathbf{A}$ were conducted to identify sources with significant group differences and, for the identified source (Fig. 8.3), the joint probability of the multimodal *data* $p(x_1(n_1), x_2(n_2))$ was assessed by means of subject-specific joint histograms.

Lastly, fusion of EEG and fMRI features (Calhoun et al. 2006c) from 23 healthy control subjects enabled an attempt to resolve neuronal source activity with both high temporal and spatial resolution without needing to directly solve hard, untractable inverse problems. Event related potentials (ERP) were generated by time-locked averaging target epochs of the EEG signals from the midline central electrode (Cz) 200ms before to 1200ms after each target stimulus in an auditory "oddball" task. Also, t-statistic maps were obtained from fitting a GLM of regression to every voxel timeseries of a BOLD fMRI scan during the same oddball task, for a target-versus-standard contrast. Both features (ERPs ($\mathbf{X}_1$) and t-statistic maps ($\mathbf{X}_2$)) were computed on the same subjects for both modalities, with ERPs being interpolated to a number of ERP timepoints (N_1) that matched the number of fMRI voxels (N_2). Joint estimation of the ERP temporal sources ($\mathbf{Y}_1$) and t-map spatial sources ($\mathbf{Y}_2$) was carried out with jICA. High temporal and spatial resolution "snapshots" were then estimated by combining the multimodal sources, first as rows of $\mathbf{F}_{N_1 \times N_2} = \left|\mathbf{Y}_1^\top\right| \mathbf{Y}_2$ (an fMRI movie at high temporal resolution—Fig. 8.4), then as rows of $\mathbf{E}_{N_2 \times N_1} = \left|\mathbf{Y}_2^\top\right| \mathbf{Y}_1$ (a set of voxel-specific ERPs at

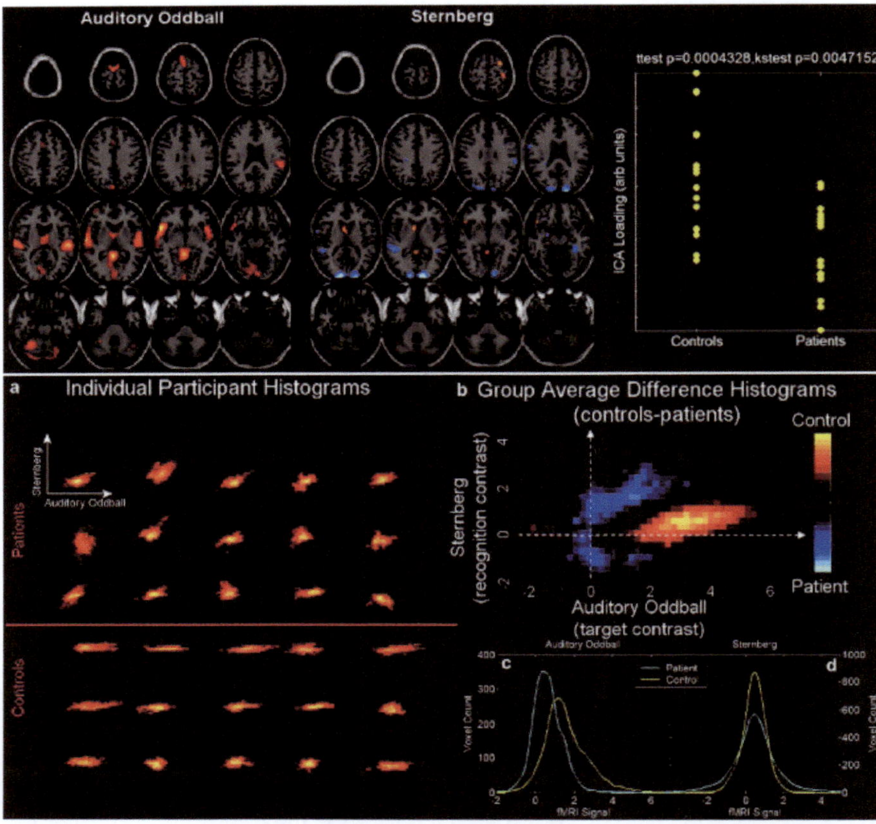

Fig. 8.2 Joint patterns of multitask group differences in schizophrenia. Top panel: Coupled joint source (network of co-varying maximally spatially independent maps) with significant difference in mixing coefficients between healthy controls and schizophrenic patients. Schizophrenia patients demonstrated lower mixing coefficient values **A** (the ICA loadings), which was interpreted as decreased functional connectivity in the joint network, particularly in temporal lobe, cerebellum, thalamus, basal ganglia, and lateral frontal regions, consistent with the cognitive dysmetria and frontotemporal disconnection models. Lower panel: (**a**) Subject-specific joint histograms: the correlation between the two tasks was significantly higher in patients than in controls, suggesting they activated "more similarly" on both tasks than controls; (**b**) Difference of group average histograms; (**c**,**d**) Marginal histograms: more AOD task voxels were active in controls and the SB task showed heavier tails in patients. Overall, the authors concluded that "patients are activating less, but also activating with a less-unique set of regions for these very different tasks." This suggested "both a global attenuation of activity as well as a breakdown of specialized wiring between cognitive domains." Copyright (2005) Wiley. Used with permission from V. D. Calhoun, *A method for multitask fMRI data fusion applied to schizophrenia*, Human Brain Mapping, John Wiley and Sons

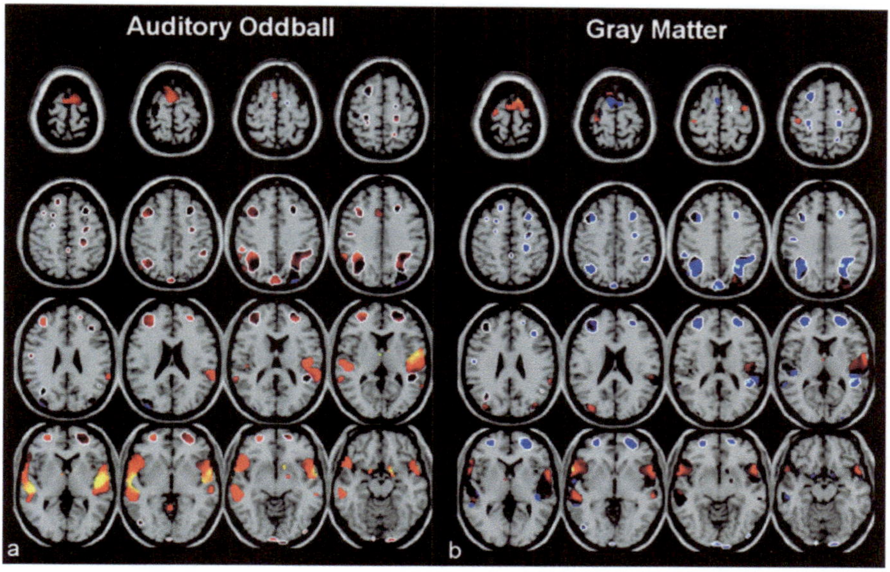

Fig. 8.3 Joint patterns of structural and functional group differences in schizophrenia. A joint multimodal independent source (not shown) with significant difference in mixing coefficients between patients and controls (higher for controls than for patients). Healthy controls showed mostly higher AOD activation in bilateral temporal lobe structures and cerebellum, associated with lower GM concentrations in bilateral frontal and parietal, as well as right temporal regions (not shown). A hypothesis of GM regions serving as "a morphological substrate for changes in AOD functional connectivity in schizophrenia" was suggested based on the coupling of those modalities via their shared mixing coefficients. The figure illustrates the t-values of a voxel-wise two-sample t-test for controls vs. patients of the data ($\mathbf{X}_1$ and $\mathbf{X}_2$) within the source regions surviving a $|Z| > 3.5$ threshold: (**a**) group differences in the AOD data over regions detected in the AOD part of the joint source (no outline) and GM part of the joint source (outlined in white), showing "more AOD activation in controls than patients." (**b**) group differences in the GM data over regions detected in the AOD part of the joint source (no outline) and GM part of the joint source (outlined in white), showing "GM values are increased in controls" over the AOD-detected regions, and decreased over the GM-detected regions (more so on the left than on the right). Orange: controls > patients; blue: the opposite. Copyright (2005) Wiley. Used with permission from V. D. Calhoun, *Method for Multimodal Analysis of Independent Source Differences in Schizophrenia: Combining Gray Matter Structural and Auditory Oddball Functional Data*, Human Brain Mapping, John Wiley and Sons

high spatial resolution—not shown), where $|\cdot|$ is the element-wise absolute value function. Overall, the results provide compelling evidence of the utility of such descriptive representation of the spatiotemporal dynamics of the auditory oddball target detection response, allowing the visualization, in humans, of the involved neural systems including participatory deep brain structures.

In summary, these results corroborate with previous evidence that methods combining the strengths of both techniques may reveal unique information and provide new insights into human brain function.

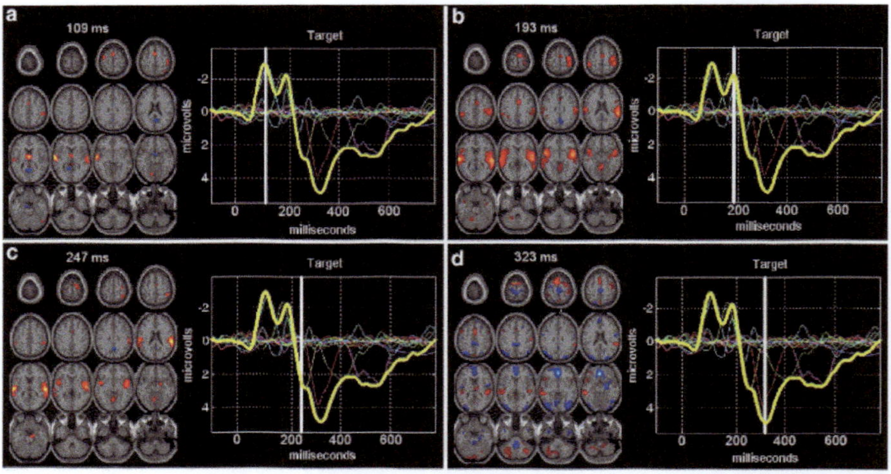

Fig. 8.4 Spatiotemporal dynamics of the auditory oddball target response. The N1 peak for the ERP data corresponded to primary and secondary auditory regions of the temporal lobe, and motor planning regions, as was expected following the initial auditory stimulus and the ensuing preparatory motor activity for the button press. Similarly, the N2 peak showed correspondence with extensive temporal lobe areas, including heteromodal association cortex, with motor planning, primary motor, and cerebellar regions also present, consistent with regions typically involved in the execution of the motor response. The P3a peak corresponded with additional temporal lobe regions, somatosensory cortex, and brain stem activity, consistent with what would be expected. In particular, the reported association of brain stem activity was evidence supportive of a previously hypothesized role for the locus coeruleus norepinephrine (LC-NE) system in generating the P3. This led to the conclusion that jICA can "reveal electrical sources which may not be readily visible to scalp ERPs and expose brain regions that have participatory roles in source activity but may not themselves be generators of the detected electrical signal." The image shows positive (orange) and negative (blue) Z values. Reprinted from NeuroImage, Vol 30 (1), V. D. Calhoun et al., *Neuronal chronometry of target detection: Fusion of hemodynamic and event-related potential data*, Pages 544–553, Copyright (2006), with permission from Elsevier

8.2.3 Advanced Blind Source Separation

The vast majority of approaches for multimodal analysis with BSS are rooted on MDU models. Their key strength is in the ability to not only utilize uncorrelation (or independence) between hidden sources for separation, like separate SDU models for each modality would do, but also leverage the correlation (or dependence) among corresponding multimodal sources to help steer the estimation procedure, automatically identifying linked sources. This increases the overall source separation power by leveraging information in one modality to improve estimation in the other modalities and vice-versa. In the following, we briefly review a number of MDU models and their applications to brain data analysis. The reader is encouraged to explore a recent review (Silva et al. 2016) which outlines further details on the models discussed below.

When (un)correlation, i.e., *linear* (in)dependence, is the sole mechanism for identification and separation of the sources, the models are categorized as second-order statistics (SOS) models. Classical algorithms such as CCA (Hotelling 1936) and PLS (Wold 1966), as well as more recent models such as multiset CCA (mCCA) (Kettenring 1971) and second-order IVA (IVA-G) (Anderson et al. 2010, 2012; Adalı et al. 2014) fall under this category. CCA maximizes the *correlation* between related source pairs $\mathbf{y}_{k=i} = [y_{1i},\ y_{2i}]^\top$ within the same subspace k, where $y_{1i} = \mathbf{W}_{1i}\mathbf{x}_1$ and $y_{2i} = \mathbf{W}_{2i}\mathbf{x}_2$ for $i = 1 \ldots C$ sources, and $\mathbf{W}_{mi}$ is the i-th row of $\mathbf{W}_m$, while PLS maximizes their *covariance* instead. Some extensions of these approaches have focused on expanding these notions beyond just 2 datasets (or modalities), like multi-set CCA (mCCA) (Correa et al. 2009), as well as leveraging higher-order statistics (HOS) to exploit source independence rather than uncorrelation, as in higher-order IVA (Anderson et al. 2013).

CCA's closed form solution for $M = 2$ datasets was utilized by Correa et al. (2008) to identify highly correlated subject expression profiles across fMRI+ERP and fMRI+sMRI datasets (with N = number of subjects). For three modalities, mCCA based on sum of squared correlations (SSQCOR) was utilized for 3-way fusion of fMRI+ERP+sMRI (Correa et al. 2009), also seeking correlated subject expression profiles. In the case of fusion of simultaneous (concurrent) fMRI+EEG, efforts have been made to identify correlated temporal profiles (N = time points) using mCCA across modalities and subjects (one downsampled, HRF-convolved single-trial ERP dataset and one fMRI dataset per subject: $M = 2 \times$ number of subjects) (Correa et al. 2010). In all cases above, the mixing matrix was estimated as $\mathbf{A}_m = \mathbf{X}\mathbf{Y}_m^-$, motivated by least squares projection. A CCA-type analysis was also pursued in source power comodulation (SPoC) (Dähne et al. 2014a), seeking associations between windowed variance profiles (neuronal oscillations from EEG) in $\mathbf{y}_1$ and a single known fixed reference source (behaviorally relevant parameters) y_{21} (considered to be already unmixed). Extensions of this method include canonical SPoC (cSPoC) (Dähne et al. 2014b), which pursued CCA between "envelope" transformations (instantaneous amplitudes) of $\mathbf{y}_m$, where $\mathbf{x}_m$ were rest EEG data from the same subject filtered at different frequency bands, and multimodal SPoC (mSPoC) (Dähne et al. 2013), which pursued CCA between simultaneously measured EEG (or MEG) temporal sources $\mathbf{y}_1$ and temporally filtered windowed variance profiles of fNIRS (or fMRI) temporal sources $\mathbf{y}_2$. The key differences between CCA and SPoC-type approaches are that $\mathbf{y}_1$ and $\mathbf{y}_2$ can have different number of observations and at least one set of sources undergoes a *non-linear* transformation. Another recent variant of CCA for multimodal fusion in neuroimaging is structured and sparse CCA (ssCCA) (Mohammadi-Nejad et al. 2017). This approach also identifies highly correlated subject expression profiles from multimodal data but imposes non-negativity, sparsity, and neighboring structure constraints on each row of $\mathbf{W}_m$. These constraints are expected to improve the interpretability of the resulting features directly from $\mathbf{W}_m$ (i.e., with no estimation of $\mathbf{A}_m$). The approach was utilized for fusion of eigenvector centrality maps of rest fMRI and T1-weighted sMRI from 34 Alzheimer's disease (AD) and 42 elderly healthy controls from the

Alzheimer's Disease Neuroimaging Initiative (ADNI) cohort, identifying two sets of multimodal regions highly associated to the disease label.

For PLS, Chen et al. (2009) utilized PLS regression to analyze GM concentration images from sMRI and ^{18}F-fluorodeoxyglucose (FDG) PET in two ways: (1) defining $\mathbf{X}_1$ as the GM maps from N subjects, $\mathbf{X}_2$ as the FDG maps from the same N subjects, and utilizing the (multivariate) PLS2 deflation strategy (Silva et al. 2016) to predict the FDG maps from the GM maps; and (2) defining $\mathbf{X}_1 = [\mathbf{X}_{FDG}^\top, \mathbf{X}_{GM}^\top]^\top$, i.e., the $(V_1 + V_2) \times N$ spatial concatenation of FDG and GM maps, and $\mathbf{X}_2$ as the $1 \times N$ age group label (younger or older), using (univariate) PLS1 for deflation (Silva et al. 2016), deflating only $\mathbf{X}_2$ (but not $\mathbf{X}_1$, for the sake of better interpretability). The latter approach is akin to jICA in the sense that the joint spatial features "share" similar expression levels over subjects, although here data reduction occurs at the feature dimension (V_m) instead of the subject dimension (N). The same approach was recently used with 3 modalities on mild cognitive impairment (MCI) patients, some of which had converted to Alzheimer's disease (AD) and some who had not (Wang et al. 2016). A similar study on a larger population is also available (Lorenzi et al. 2016).

In the case of modalities whose data can be arranged into multidimensional arrays, it is possible to utilize multilinear algebra to extend PLS into multi-way[1] PLS (N-PLS). This was utilized to fuse simultaneous EEG and fMRI recordings of subjects resting with eyes closed (Martínez-Montes et al. 2004). The data was organized into a 3-way tensor $\mathbf{X}_1$ with the $V_1 \times N \times D$ EEG data and a matrix (2-way tensor) $\mathbf{X}_2$ with the $V_2 \times N$ fMRI data, where N was the number of timepoints (and corresponding EEG 'segments'), V_1 was the number of frequencies in the EEG spectrum of each EEG segment, V_2 was the number of fMRI voxels, and D was the number of EEG electrode channels. For the EEG data, the frequencies of each electrode were convolved with the HRF over the time dimension to yield temporal "envelopes" of the EEG signal that were comparable to the fMRI timeseries. The model used for the EEG tensor was equivalent to $\mathbf{X}_{1,d} = \mathbf{A}_1\text{diag}(\mathbf{b}_d)\mathbf{Y}_1$, $d = 1, \ldots, D$, where $\text{diag}(\mathbf{b}_d)$ is a diagonal matrix with $\mathbf{b}_d$ in the diagonal, i.e., the same decomposition $\mathbf{A}_1\mathbf{Y}_1$ was estimated in every EEG channel except for a set of scaling values $\mathbf{b}_d$ specific to each channel, which can be interpreted as a model of shared (i.e., same) sources $\mathbf{Y}_1$ with electrode-specific mixing $\mathbf{A}_{1,d} = \mathbf{A}_1\text{diag}(\mathbf{b}_d)$. The covariance between the temporal EEG envelope sources $\mathbf{Y}_1$ and fMRI time course sources $\mathbf{Y}_2$ was then maximized, utilizing an extension of the PLS2 deflation strategy, which accommodates tensors, to predict the fMRI timeseries $\mathbf{X}_2$ from the EEG envelope sources $\mathbf{Y}_1$. This procedure yielded an fMRI map (a column of $\mathbf{A}_2$) whose time course (row of $\mathbf{Y}_2$) covaried highly with an EEG envelope (row of $\mathbf{Y}_1$) corresponding to an alpha band spectrum (column of $\mathbf{A}_1$) and a topographical map described by the electrode-specific scalars $\mathbf{b}_d$. This topographical map was

[1]While here "multi-way" refers to the order of a tensor (i.e., the number of data dimensions), the term multi-way has also been used in the literature to refer to the number of modalities being fused.

also studied using current source localization to identify the generators of the "EEG alpha rhythm".

For IVA, in comparison to mCCA, there are two key differences: (1) **W** is not constrained to have orthogonal rows,[2] and (2) HOS can be utilized to identify the sources. Together, these differences allow IVA to generalize mCCA, attaining more compact representations in **A** (Adalı et al. 2015) and leveraging HOS *dependence* between linked sources for improved separation.[3] Moreover, in a comparison with jICA, Adalı et al. (2015) noted that although IVA is more flexible when the subject expression profiles differ across a subset of the datasets (i.e., when the "same mixing matrix" assumption of jICA is violated), in very small N (number of subjects) regimes HOS estimation is unreliable and, thus, infeasible. Therefore, IVA-G was utilized instead, since it relies exclusively on SOS, just like mCCA. In the study, a GLM contrast map from fMRI, a GM concentration map from sMRI, and an ERP timeseries from EEG were obtained from 22 healthy controls and 14 schizophrenic patients ($N = 36$ subjects) performing an AOD task. Results from single and pairwise combinations of modalities were compared against the three-modality case. The study concluded that, for this particularly small dataset, "jICA provides a more desirable solution" using a flexible density matching ICA algorithm, a result likely driven by the drastically larger number of observations in the jICA model versus that of IVA for this study.

Another class of data fusion algorithms is based on two-step approaches that pursue BSS of either **A** or **Y** separately, after fitting an initial BSS model on **X**. Two models that stand out in this class are "spatial" CCA+jICA (Sui et al. 2010) and mCCA+jICA (Sui et al. 2011). Spatial CCA+jICA uses CCA to initially identify correlated sources $\mathbf{Y}_1^{\text{CCA}} = \mathbf{W}_1^{\text{CCA}}\mathbf{X}_1$ and $\mathbf{Y}_2^{\text{CCA}} = \mathbf{W}_2^{\text{CCA}}\mathbf{X}_2$ in the usual way. However, within each modality, these CCA sources are just uncorrelated, and their separation is not guaranteed if the underlying source (canonical) correlations are equal or very similar (Sui et al. 2010). Thus, jICA on the concatenated *source* matrices $\mathbf{Y}_1^{\text{CCA}}$ and $\mathbf{Y}_2^{\text{CCA}}$ is utilized to further identify joint *independent* sources $\mathbf{Y}_1^{\text{jICA}} = \mathbf{W}^{\text{jICA}}\mathbf{Y}_1^{\text{CCA}}$ and $\mathbf{Y}_2^{\text{jICA}} = \mathbf{W}^{\text{jICA}}\mathbf{Y}_2^{\text{CCA}}$, where $\mathbf{W}^{\text{jICA}}$ is shared across modalities. The final mixing matrix of the spatial CCA+jICA model is then estimated as $\mathbf{A}_m = \left(\mathbf{W}^{\text{jICA}}\mathbf{W}_m^{\text{CCA}}\right)^{-}$. This model was utilized on multitask fMRI contrast maps derived from subject-level GLM (see Sect. 8.2.2), with $V =$ subjects and $N =$ feature dimensionality (here, voxels), resulting in interpretable multitask independent sources with similar (i.e. highly correlated) spatial map configurations (Sui et al. 2010). To note, such property should also be attainable with IVA directly applied to $\mathbf{X}_m$ and is worth of further investigation. The mCCA+jICA approach (Sui et al. 2011), on the other hand, utilizes mCCA to initially identify highly correlated *subject expression profiles* (rather than features) across m

[2] IVA-G is identical to mCCA with the GENVAR cost, except it also allows non-orthogonal **W**.

[3] The IVA cost is a sum of M separate ICAs (one per dataset) with an additional term to increase/retain the mutual information between corresponding sources across datasets.

modalities, $\mathbf{Y}_{\mathrm{CCA},m}^{\top} = \mathbf{X}_m \mathbf{W}_{\mathrm{CCA},m}^{\top}$, where $\mathbf{X}_m$ is $V \times N_m$ (number of subjects (V) by feature dimensionality (N_m)). Notice the multiplication from the right of $\mathbf{X}_m$ and the matrix transposes resulting from V being treated as the observations. Thus, the mCCA $V \times N_m$ mixing matrices constitute the features estimated by least squares as $\mathbf{A}_{\mathrm{CCA},m}^{\top} = (\mathbf{Y}_{\mathrm{CCA},m}^{\top})^{-}\mathbf{X}_m$. Joint ICA is then performed on the concatenated *mixing matrices* $\mathbf{A}_{\mathrm{CCA},m}^{\top}$ (along the feature dimension N_m) to identify joint sources $\mathbf{Y}_{\mathrm{jICA},m} = \mathbf{W}_{\mathrm{jICA}} \mathbf{A}_{\mathrm{CCA},m}^{\top}$, where the $V \times V$ matrix $\mathbf{W}_{\mathrm{jICA}}$ is shared across modalities. The final mixing matrix of the mCCA+jICA model is then estimated as $\mathbf{A}_m = \mathbf{Y}_{\mathrm{CCA},m}^{\top} \mathbf{W}_{\mathrm{jICA}}^{-1}$. This model was used by Sui et al. (2011) to perform fusion of GLM-derived fMRI contrast maps and DWI fractional anisotropy (FA) maps from each subject, yielding good separation across 62 healthy control (HC), 54 schizophrenic (SZ), and 48 bipolar (BP) disorder subjects, as indicated by pair-wise two-sample t-tests of the group mixing coefficients in each column of each $\mathbf{A}_m$. Source maps for each group and modality were obtained by back-reconstruction, partitioning $\mathbf{A}_m$ into three blocks, $\mathbf{A}_{g,m}$, $g \in \{\mathrm{HC}, \mathrm{SZ}, \mathrm{BP}\}$, one from each group respectively, and computing $\mathbf{Y}_{g,m} = (\mathbf{A}_{g,m})^{-}\mathbf{X}_{g,m}$. In a 3-way study, Sui et al. (2013) explored this approach to study group differences between 116 healthy controls and 97 schizophrenic patients, fusing GLM-derived contrast maps for the tapping condition of a block-design auditory sensorimotor task, together with FA maps and GM concentration maps from each subject. Finally, a very large study by Miller et al. (2016) on $V = 5{,}034$ subjects from the UK Biobank cohort defined $\mathbf{X}_1$ as a collection of $N_1 = 2{,}501$ image-derived phenotype (IDP) variables (individual measures of brain structure from T1-, T2-, and susceptibility-weighted sMRI, brain activity from task and rest fMRI, and local tissue microstructure from diffusion MRI), and $\mathbf{X}_2$ as a collection of $N_2 = 1{,}100$ non-imaging phenotype (non-IDP) variables extracted from the UK Biobank database (grouped into 11 categories) on the same subjects. In this study, the subject expression profiles were combined into a single *shared* profile, $\mathbf{Y}_{\mathrm{CCA}}^{\top} = \mathbf{Y}_{\mathrm{CCA},1}^{\top} + \mathbf{Y}_{\mathrm{CCA},2}^{\top}$, which was used to estimate the modality-specific CCA mixing matrices, i.e., the features[4] $\mathbf{A}_{\mathrm{CCA},m}^{\top} = (\mathbf{Y}_{\mathrm{CCA}}^{\top})^{-}\mathbf{X}_m$. Moreover, rather than estimating mixing matrices with the form above, a final *shared* mixing matrix of the mCCA+jICA model is estimated as $\mathbf{A} = \mathbf{Y}_{\mathrm{CCA}}^{\top} \mathbf{A}_{\mathrm{jICA}}$, where $\mathbf{A}_{\mathrm{jICA}} = \left[\mathbf{A}_{\mathrm{CCA},1}^{\top}, \mathbf{A}_{\mathrm{CCA},2}^{\top}\right] \cdot \left[\mathbf{Y}_{\mathrm{jICA},1}, \mathbf{Y}_{\mathrm{jICA},2}\right]^{-}$ ($[\,\cdot\,,\,\cdot\,]$ indicates matrix concatenation).[5]

[4]The MATLAB code used for this study (available at http://www.fmrib.ox.ac.uk/ukbiobank/nnpaper/ukb_NN.m) actually implements this step as $\left[\mathbf{A}_{\mathrm{CCA},1}, \mathbf{A}_{\mathrm{CCA},2}\right] = F(\mathbf{R}^{\mathbf{yx}})$, where $F(\cdot) = \mathrm{atanh}(\cdot)$ is the element-wise Fisher transform of the $C \times (N_1 + N_2)$ cross-correlation matrix $\mathbf{R}^{\mathbf{yx}} = \mathrm{diag}\left(\mathbf{Y}_{\mathrm{CCA}}\mathbf{Y}_{\mathrm{CCA}}^{\top}\right)^{-\frac{1}{2}} (\mathbf{Y}_{\mathrm{CCA}}\mathbf{X})\mathrm{diag}\left(\mathbf{X}^{\top}\mathbf{X}\right)^{-\frac{1}{2}}$ between $\mathbf{y}_{\mathrm{CCA}}$ and $\mathbf{x}^{\top}$, $\mathrm{diag}(\mathbf{B})$ is a diagonal matrix containing only the diagonal elements of $\mathbf{B}$, and $\mathbf{X} = [\mathbf{X}_1, \mathbf{X}_2]$ is a matrix concatenation. Equivalence to the form indicated in the main text is claimed but not proven.

[5]Note that the implementation of mCCA+jICA in that work utilized simple matrix transpose instead of the pseudo-inverses indicted above, possibly presuming that the columns of $\mathbf{Y}_{\mathrm{CCA}}^{\top}$ and rows of $\left[\mathbf{Y}_{\mathrm{jICA},1}, \mathbf{Y}_{\mathrm{jICA},2}\right]$ are orthonormal due to uncorrelation and independence, respectively.

Finally, approaches such as Parallel ICA (Liu et al. 2007) make up a unique class of BSS methods that seek to attain multiple goals simultaneously in an adaptive fashion. Specifically, rather than pursuing a decomposition into two sequential steps like with mCCA+jICA, Parallel ICA carries out separate ICA decompositions of each modality (i.e., in "parallel") while simultaneously identifying and reinforcing associations (in the form of correlations) among specific rows/columns of $\mathbf{A}_m$, $\mathbf{Y}_m$, or both, depending on how the modalities are treated/organized (i.e., if one or more of the datasets is transposed or not). The most widely used implementation simultaneously optimizes for maximal independence among sources $\mathbf{y}_m$ for each modality, treating the columns of $\mathbf{Y}_m$ as observations (like multiple separate SDU models), and maximal correlation among corresponding *mixing coefficients* $\mathbf{a}_k = [a_{1k}, a_{2k}, \ldots, a_{Mk}]^{\top}$ over modalities, treating the rows of $\mathbf{A}_m$ as observations (like an MDU model, but operating on pair-wise correlations individually rather than as a cohesive correlation matrix). These are typically competing objectives, leading to a trade-off between them (Vergara et al. 2014). Parallel ICA has been widely used in imaging genetics, offering a direct approach to identify neuroimaging endophenotypes related to various mental illnesses by fusing modalities such as fMRI and SNP (Liu et al. 2009), sMRI and SNP (Meda et al. 2012), as well as fMRI, sMRI, and SNP in a 3-way analysis (Vergara et al. 2014). It has also found use in fusion of resting-state networks (RSN) and behavioral measures (Meier et al. 2012).

While BSS has proven to be very fruitful for multimodal fusion thus far, it has mostly been focused on MDU methods. Much stands to be gained from subspaces that span multiple sources within a single dataset in terms of both improved representation power of complex features and, especially, subject-specific characterizations. Such MDM approaches are poised to move multimodal fusion analyses much further and address some of the current challenges and limitations of the area. Indeed, MDM models can be seen as two-layer-deep multimodal networks with fixed connections at the second layer. Thus, one interpretation of MDM models is that they have the ability to recover certain non-linear mixtures of the sources. Given the nature of complex systems such as the brain, sources are highly likely to be non-linearly mixed, which also serves as motivation to the deep learning methods described in Sect. 8.3.

8.2.4 Further Reading

For a unifying BSS modeling framework and discourse on the connections between various additional BSS methods applied to multimodal and unimodal brain imaging data, see Silva et al. (2016).

For a general review on multimodal fusion for brain imaging data, see Calhoun and Sui (2016).

For an overview of methods, challenges, and prospects of multimodal fusion beyond the scope of brain imaging, see Lahat et al. (2015).

For a broader discussion of methods beyond BSS and their application to multimodal brain imaging integration, see Biessmann et al. (2011).

For a clear, generalized description of tensor analysis and fusion as coupled matrix-tensor factorization methods, see Karahan et al. (2015).

For a comprehensive and mathematically oriented account of SDU models, see the Handbook of BSS (Comon and Jutten 2010).

Finally, the less experienced reader interested in a smooth introduction to the preprocessing strategies leading into ICA (and beyond) are recommended to check out the excellent ICA book from Hyvärinen et al. (2002). Those readers might also enjoy the numerous insights contained in the chapter about methods grounded on information theory (including ICA) by Haykin (2008).

8.3 Deep Learning Methods

In the previous section we presented blind source separation approaches in the context of multimodal fusion, particularly those based on MDU models, which may be construed as items of a more general area of *unsupervised learning*. Naturally, the models considered thus far utilize only a single level of *linear* transformation of sources (for generation) or data (for decomposition). However, if deeper chains of linear transformations are considered, each followed by a *nonlinear activation function* of its outputs (Goodfellow et al. 2016), much more powerful and flexible models can be obtained, naturally allowing compositions of multiple modalities, all while resorting to just simple stochastic gradient descent (SGD) for optimization (Goodfellow et al. 2016, Section 8.3.1). While these deeper models are able to approximate arbitrarily complex nonlinearities in the data, simple SOS or HOS does not suffice to attain the typical "blind" property that is characteristic of *linear* BSS (Comon and Jutten 2010, Chapter 14). Thus, for the purposes of this section, we forfeit this property in favor of *supervised* deep models, which, in neuroimaging, constitute the majority of successful deep learning results obtained from real multimodal brain imaging data.

Feedforward Neural Networks, or multilayer perceptrons (MLPs), are a classic model for function approximation, such as for classifiers, where $\mathbf{y} = \mathbf{G}(\mathbf{x})$ maps an input data sample $\mathbf{x}$ to output labels $\mathbf{y}$. The mapping $\mathbf{G}(\cdot)$ can be approximated by an L-layer network $\mathbf{g}(\mathbf{x}, \boldsymbol{\Phi}) = \mathbf{g}^L(\mathbf{g}^{L-1}(\cdots(\mathbf{g}^1(\mathbf{x}))))$ with parameters $\boldsymbol{\Phi}$. Each function $\mathbf{g}^l$ is defined as a linear model $\mathbf{W}_l\mathbf{g}^{l-1} + b_l$, with weights $\mathbf{W}_l$ and bias b_l, followed by nonlinear functions $\mathbf{h}$ (the activation functions), such that:

$$\mathbf{g}^l = \mathbf{h}(\mathbf{W}_l\mathbf{g}^{l-1} + b_l), \tag{8.1}$$

where $\mathbf{g}^0 = \mathbf{x}$, and $\boldsymbol{\Phi} = \{\mathbf{W}_l, b_l \; ; \; l = 1 \ldots L\}$.

In the case of the increasingly popular *convolutional neural networks* (CNNs), instead of a matrix multiplication $\mathbf{W}_l\mathbf{x}$, convolution with some kernel $\mathbf{W}_l$ is utilized at each layer:

$$\mathbf{g}^l = \mathbf{h}(\mathbf{W}_l * \mathbf{g}^{l-1} + b_l). \tag{8.2}$$

In this case, it is common to also define $\mathbf{g}^l$ at certain layers as other operations such as pooling, for example "max pooling" (Zhou and Chellappa 1988), normalization, for example batch normalization (Ioffe and Szegedy 2015), or dropout (Srivastava et al. 2014).

CNNs have multiple advantages (Goodfellow et al. 2016) over MLPs when the input data contains local correlations. CNNs exploit that with their local and, as such, sparse connections. If in MLPs we are connecting every input with every output, here we are applying a kernel to only a small region of input defined by the kernel size. Yet, in deeper layers, neurons are still indirectly connected to larger regions of the input. The size of the region a neuron connects to within its input layer is determined by the size of its receptive field, which depends on the CNN's hyperparameters and architecture. Overall, local connectivity reduces the number of parameters, computational complexity and memory requirements. All that is achieved via parameter-tying, i.e., when the same parameters are (re)used for multiple locations of the input. Furthermore, convolving the same parameter kernel with the input yields translation invariance property of images.

When the CNN is used as a classifier, in which use it has arguably revived increased interest to neural networks and started the ongoing deep learning revolution (Krizhevsky et al. 2012), then the convolutional layers are followed by a few feed forward layers with the softmax prediction at the end. However, for some applications, such as segmentation, it is preferable to stay within convolution layers only and in this case the network is called fully convolutional (Long et al. 2015)

Both CNN types are shown in Fig. 8.5 and in the following sections we will give a short overview of the use of these models.

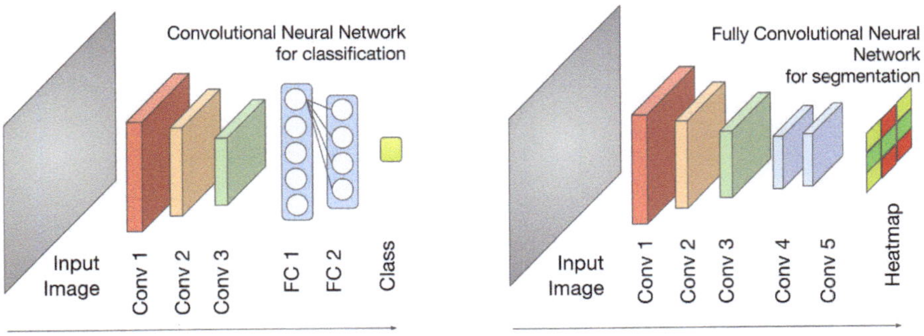

Fig. 8.5 Convolutional and fully convolutional neural networks. When used for classification tasks, CNNs typically feed directly into fully connected (FC) layers before classification. In segmentation tasks, however, fully convolutional networks can better retain the spatial structure of the data

8.3.1 Multimodal Classification

Feed forward neural networks are powerful classifiers that can achieve superior accuracy when trained on representative data. Their flexible and extensible architecture can be adjusted to handle cases that arise in practice. Ulloa et al. (2018) have built a multimodal classifier which combines structural and functional data to predict schizophrenia from brain imaging data (see Fig. 8.6). However, typical brain imaging datasets are comprised of fairly small numbers of subjects. To overcome the large data size requirements for training deep models, synthetic data generation approaches based on SDU models such as ICA have been proposed for augmenting these small datasets (Castro et al. 2015; Ulloa et al. 2015). Expanding on this idea, Ulloa et al. (2018) proposed to augment the training sets of datasets originating from different modalities. The augmentation process involves training a spatial ICA model for each modality (N = number of voxels) to learn both mixings $\mathbf{A}_m$ and sources $\mathbf{Y}_m$. Then, using only the labels of the training set, multidimensional sampling generates multiple new instances of mixing matrices $\mathbf{A}_m^r$ similar to $\mathbf{A}_m$. These are then combined with the ICA estimated sources $\mathbf{Y}_m$ to generate new synthetic examples of labeled data $\mathbf{X}_m^r$.

Initially, deep MLPs were trained separately for each modality utilizing only the synthetic data $\mathbf{X}_m^r$. The weights $\mathbf{W}_l$ from each MLP were then utilized to initialize the modality-specific weights of the final multimodal MLP, as indicated in Fig. 8.6. The multimodal MLP was then trained only on real data to classify disease labels using cross-validation. The resulting trained network was then evaluated on the test set in a 10-fold cross validation procedure yielding significantly improved results over other state of the art models, including the same MLP, that were either trained on a single modality or without using synthetic data (see Table 8.1).

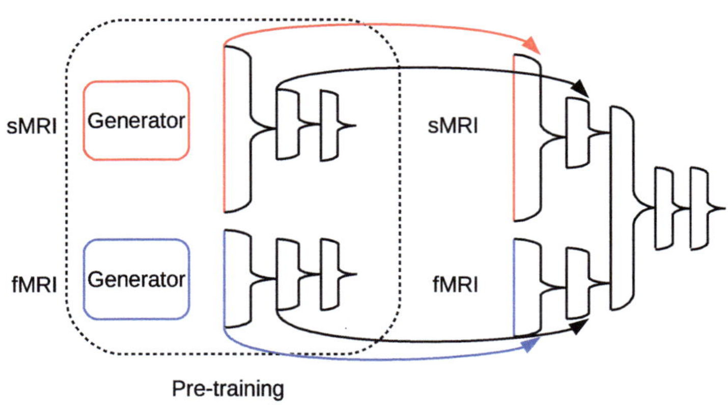

Fig. 8.6 Multimodal classifier. A multimodal MLP is one in which the deeper layers of the unimodal networks are combined (concatenated) together and treated as one. Here, the unimodal networks were trained on synthetic data separately. The weights learned on each modality separately using synthetic data were utilized to initialize the weights of the combined multimodal network, which was then trained using only real data

Table 8.1 Average and standard deviation of the area under the ROC curve (AUC) of an 8-fold cross validation experiment for various classifiers and the proposed methodologies

	sMRI		fMRI		sMRI + fMRI	
Classifier Method	Average AUC	Standard deviation	Average AUC	Standard deviation	Average AUC	Standard deviation
Online learning and synthetic data						
MLP with MVN	0.65	0.05	0.82	0.06	**0.85**	**0.05**
MLP with rejection	**0.74**	**0.07**	**0.83**	**0.05**	0.84	0.05
Raw data						
MLP	0.65	0.09	0.82	0.10	0.80	0.08
Naive Bayes	0.62	0.10	0.71	0.11	0.61	0.07
Logistic Regression	0.69	0.12	0.82	0.07	0.81	0.08
RBF SVM	0.53	0.05	0.82	0.08	0.58	0.15
Linear SVM	0.68	0.09	0.82	0.06	0.80	0.15
LDA	0.73	0.10	0.79	0.09	0.79	0.11
Random Forest	0.65	0.06	0.64	0.05	0.67	0.08
Nearest Neighbors	0.58	0.07	0.68	0.08	0.61	0.12
Decision Tree	0.56	0.11	0.54	0.10	0.53	0.13

8.3.2 Representation Learning for Semantic Embedding

The predictive advantages of multilayered models such as feed forward neural networks come from the powerful representations of the data that they automatically obtain at training. What that means is that the network learns a mapping of input data to the output layer vector space, where the input data samples are easily separable, thus encoding regularities in the data that are not easy to specify upfront. These output layer embeddings can be visualized if the multidimensional vectors are "projected" to a 2D space. Simple linear projections usually do not work well for this purpose, but nonlinear embedding methods such as t-distributed stochastic neighbor embedding (tSNE) (Maaten and Hinton 2008) do.

To obtain an embedding of a set of MRI images one first trains a deep model either for prediction or reconstruction. The obtained model is then used to produce activations at the output layer (or the one prior), which are subsequently represented as points on a 2D plane. Importantly, these points can later be assigned pseudo-color according to any property of interest. Plis et al. (2014) was one of the first to produce individual subject embeddings for MRI data. A deep 3-layer model trained to predict patients from healthy controls, possessing just that information, also learned to segregate disease severity of the patients as shown by the yellow-red spectrum in Fig. 8.7b.

The same approach has been applied to data from the Bipolar-Schizophrenia Network on Intermediate Phenotypes consortium (B-SNIP, http://www.b-snip.org/). The network was trained to predict three diseases from the spectrum (schizophrenia, the most severe, bipolar, and schizo-affective disorders) from healthy controls. After training, this network was used to produce embeddings for the data of subjects from

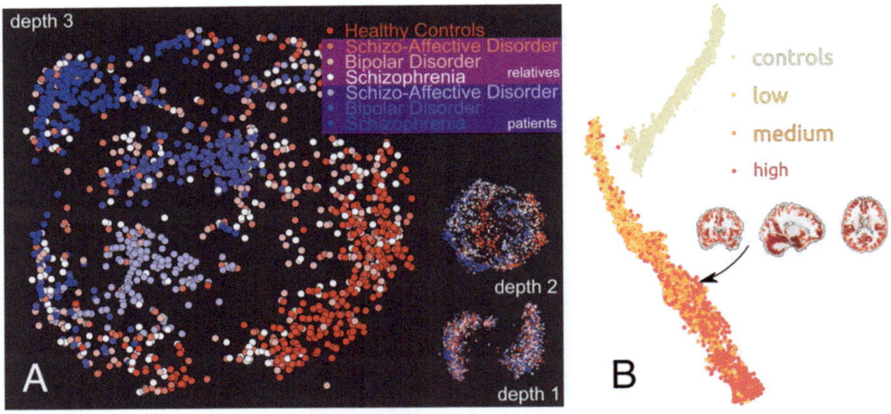

Fig. 8.7 Embedding deep network representations for healthy controls, patients with a spectrum of mental disorders and their unaffected siblings (**a**); for healthy controls and Huntington disease (HD) patients (**b**). Panel (**a**) also demonstrates sensitivity of embeddings to the network depth, where with depth the embedding becomes more interpretable. In panel (**b**), note the emergence of severity spectrum for HD patients despite unavailability of that information to the deep learning algorithm

its training set as well as the unaffected relatives that were previously unseen (shown in Fig. 8.7a). To further illustrate the value of depth in these models, Fig. 8.7a shows embeddings obtained from models of smaller depth: 1 and 2. These do not show such clear segregation spectrum.

8.3.3 Multimodal Tissue Segmentation

The problem of brain tissue segmentation is fundamental to almost any research study on the brain as gray matter volumes and thicknesses are potentially strong biomarkers for a number of disorders. In order to compute these, one needs to first segment the MRI images into various tissue types. Traditionally, a lengthy and computationally heavy process performed in multiple packages and usually relying on multiple sub-stages including skull stripping to rid anything but the brain. Simple gray, white matter and CSF segmentation is widespread enough to be interesting. It can sometimes be completed using simple techniques based on pixel intensity property. However, a much more valuable and yet much harder segmentation is into functional atlases, where each cortical and subcortical region is delineated according to their function relative to some atlas. The problem is challenging as it requires regions to be outlined not just based on voxel intensities alone but also on the relative location of the region within the brain.

Fedorov et al. (2017a) have successfully used a fully convolutional network of a specific kind (dilated convolutional kernels) to quickly (under 3 min, compared to more than 10 h state-of-the-art FreeSurfer (Dale et al. 1999)) partition an MRI in

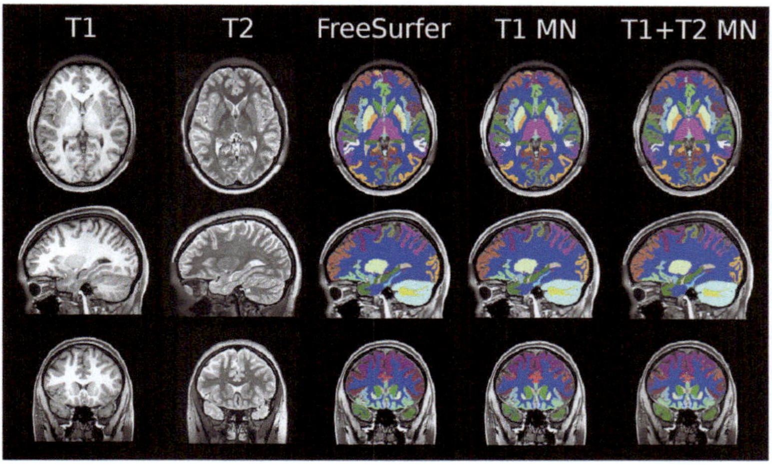

Fig. 8.8 Accelerating conventional approaches to tissue segmentation. Segmentation results produced by FreeSurfer on a single-subject image (center) after 10h of intense processing, using a trained CNN with dilated convolutional kernels (center-right) after 3 min, and using both T1 and T2 contrasts (right). T1 and T2 images included for reference (left and center-left, respectively)

the subject space into tissue types (Fedorov et al. 2017b) and functional regions. What is important for us here is that they have found significant improvements in segmentation accuracy when using multimodal input: not just T1 but also T2 contrast images (see Fig. 8.8). Deep learning models provide very simple mechanisms to use multimodal data without any additional difficulties. Another powerful feature for segmentation models comes from the fact that the learning signal can be produced at each predicted voxel, thus producing significant amounts of training data and reducing sample requirements for training. Çiçek et al. (2016) used just a handful of MRIs to produce a solid model.

8.4 Closing Remarks

Multimodal fusion is indeed a key element for discovery, understanding, and prediction in neuroimaging and mental health. Blind source separation and deep learning approaches have both demonstrated evidence of their ability to recover relevant information from multimodal data in multiple settings. The results presented here support the utility of multimodal approaches for brain imaging data analysis and suggest continued development of these methods, combined with increasingly large datasets, can yield strong, predictive features for both research and clinical settings. In particular, we highlight the current development of MDM approaches for identifying non-trivial hidden subspace structures, as well as deep architectures for unraveling the complex relationships between function and structure in the human brain. The combination of these two strategies holds great promise towards a unified approach for studying both healthy and disease conditions.

Acknowledgements We would like to thank Dr. Vince Calhoun for the useful discussions, as well as Alvaro Ulloa and Aleksandr Fedorov for kindly providing some of the images and results presented here. This work was supported by NIH grants R01EB006841 (SP), 2R01EB005846 (RS), and R01EB020407 (RS), NSF grants IIS-1318759 (SP), 1539067 (RS), and NIH NIGMS Center of Biomedical Research Excellent (COBRE) grant 5P20RR021938/P20GM103472/P30GM122734.

References

Adalı T, Anderson M, Fu GS (2014) Diversity in independent component and vector analyses: Identifiability, algorithms, and applications in medical imaging. IEEE Signal Process Mag 31(3):18–33. https://doi.org/10.1109/MSP.2014.2300511

Adalı T, Levin-Schwartz Y, Calhoun VD (2015) Multimodal data fusion using source separation: Application to medical imaging. Proc IEEE 103(9):1494–1506. https://doi.org/10.1109/JPROC.2015.2461601

Anderson M, Li XL, Adalı T (2010) Nonorthogonal independent vector analysis using multivariate gaussian model. In: Vigneron V, Zarzoso V, Moreau E, Gribonval R, Vincent E (eds) Proc LVA/ICA 2010, Lecture Notes in Computer Science, vol 6365. Springer, St. Malo, France, pp 354–361. https://doi.org/10.1007/978-3-642-15995-4_44

Anderson M, Adalı T, Li XL (2012) Joint blind source separation with multivariate gaussian model: Algorithms and performance analysis. IEEE Trans Signal Process 60(4):1672–1683. https://doi.org/10.1109/TSP.2011.2181836

Anderson M, Fu GS, Phlypo R, Adalı T (2013) Independent vector analysis, the Kotz distribution, and performance bounds. In: Proc IEEE ICASSP 2013, Vancouver, BC, pp 3243–3247. https://doi.org/10.1109/ICASSP.2013.6638257

Bell A, Sejnowski T (1995) An information-maximization approach to blind separation and blind deconvolution. Neural Comput 7(6):1129–1159

Belouchrani A, Abed-Meraim K, Cardoso JF, Moulines E (1993) Second-order blind separation of temporally correlated sources. In: Proc ICDSP 1993, Nicosia, Cyprus, pp 346–351

Biessmann F, Plis S, Meinecke FC, Eichele T, Muller KR (2011) Analysis of multimodal neuroimaging data. IEEE Rev Biomed Eng 4:26–58. https://doi.org/10.1109/RBME.2011.2170675

Calhoun VD, Adalı T (2009) Feature-based fusion of medical imaging data. IEEE Trans Inf Technol Biomed 13(5):711–720. https://doi.org/10.1109/TITB.2008.923773

Calhoun VD, Sui J (2016) Multimodal fusion of brain imaging data: A key to finding the missing link(s) in complex mental illness. Biol Psychiatry Cogn Neurosci Neuroimaging 1(3):230–244. https://doi.org/10.1016/j.bpsc.2015.12.005

Calhoun VD, Adalı T, Giuliani NR, Pekar JJ, Kiehl KA, Pearlson GD (2006a) Method for multimodal analysis of independent source differences in schizophrenia: Combining gray matter structural and auditory oddball functional data. Hum Brain Mapp 27(1):47–62. https://doi.org/10.1002/hbm.20166

Calhoun VD, Adalı T, Kiehl K, Astur R, Pekar J, Pearlson G (2006b) A method for multi-task fMRI data fusion applied to schizophrenia. Hum Brain Mapp 27(7):598–610. https://doi.org/10.1002/hbm.20204

Calhoun VD, Adalı T, Pearlson GD, Kiehl KA (2006c) Neuronal chronometry of target detection: Fusion of hemodynamic and event-related potential data. NeuroImage 30(2):544–553. https://doi.org/10.1016/j.neuroimage.2005.08.060

Cardoso JF (1998) Multidimensional independent component analysis. In: Proc IEEE ICASSP 1998, Seattle, WA, vol 4, pp 1941–1944. https://doi.org/10.1109/ICASSP.1998.681443

Castro E, Ulloa A, Plis SM, Turner JA, Calhoun VD (2015) Generation of synthetic structural magnetic resonance images for deep learning pre-training. In: Proc IEEE ISBI 2015, pp 1057–1060. https://doi.org/10.1109/ISBI.2015.7164053

Chen K, Reiman EM, Huan Z, Caselli RJ, Bandy D, Ayutyanont N, Alexander GE (2009) Linking functional and structural brain images with multivariate network analyses: A novel application of the partial least square method. NeuroImage 47(2):602–610. https://doi.org/10.1016/j.neuroimage.2009.04.053

Çiçek Ö, Abdulkadir A, Lienkamp SS, Brox T, Ronneberger O (2016) 3D U-Net: learning dense volumetric segmentation from sparse annotation. In: Proc MICCAI 2016, pp 424–432. https://doi.org/10.1007/978-3-319-46723-8_49

Comon P (1994) Independent component analysis, a new concept? Signal Process 36(3):287–314. https://doi.org/10.1016/0165-1684(94)90029-9

Comon P, Jutten C (2010) Handbook of blind source separation, 1st edn. Academic Press, Oxford, UK

Correa NM, Li YO, Adalı T, Calhoun VD (2008) Canonical correlation analysis for feature-based fusion of biomedical imaging modalities and its application to detection of associative networks in schizophrenia. IEEE J Sel Topics Signal Process 2(6):998–1007. https://doi.org/10.1109/JSTSP.2008.2008265

Correa NM, Li YO, Adalı T, Calhoun VD (2009) Fusion of fMRI, sMRI, and EEG data using canonical correlation analysis. In: Proc IEEE ICASSP 2009, pp 385–388. https://doi.org/10.1109/ICASSP.2009.4959601

Correa NM, Eichele T, Adalı T, Li YO, Calhoun VD (2010) Multi-set canonical correlation analysis for the fusion of concurrent single trial ERP and functional MRI. Neuroimage 50(4):1438–1445. https://doi.org/10.1016/j.neuroimage.2010.01.062

Dähne S, Bießmann F, Meinecke F, Mehnert J, Fazli S, Müller KR (2013) Integration of multivariate data streams with bandpower signals. IEEE Trans Multimedia 15(5):1001–1013. https://doi.org/10.1109/TMM.2013.2250267

Dähne S, Meinecke F, Haufe S, Höhne J, Tangermann M, Müller KR, Nikulin V (2014a) SPoC: A novel framework for relating the amplitude of neuronal oscillations to behaviorally relevant parameters. NeuroImage 86:111–122. https://doi.org/10.1016/j.neuroimage.2013.07.079

Dähne S, Nikulin V, Ramírez D, Schreier P, Müller KR, Haufe S (2014b) Finding brain oscillations with power dependencies in neuroimaging data. NeuroImage 96:334–348. https://doi.org/10.1016/j.neuroimage.2014.03.075

Dale AM, Fischl B, Sereno MI (1999) Cortical surface-based analysis: I. segmentation and surface reconstruction. NeuroImage 9(2):179–194. https://doi.org/10.1006/nimg.1998.0395

Fedorov A, Damaraju E, Calhoun V, Plis S (2017a) Almost instant brain atlas segmentation for large-scale studies. arXiv preprint URL http://arxiv.org/abs/1711.00457

Fedorov A, Johnson J, Damaraju E, Ozerin A, Calhoun V, Plis S (2017b) End-to-end learning of brain tissue segmentation from imperfect labeling. In: Proc IJCNN 2017, pp 3785–3792. https://doi.org/10.1109/IJCNN.2017.7966333

Goodfellow I, Bengio Y, Courville A (2016) Deep learning. MIT Press. http://www.deeplearningbook.org

Haykin S (2008) Neural networks and learning machines, 3rd edn. Prentice Hall, Upper Saddle River, NJ

Hotelling H (1936) Relations between two sets of variates. Biometrika 28(3/4):321–377. https://doi.org/10.2307/2333955

Hyvärinen A, Erkki O (1997) A fast fixed-point algorithm for independent component analysis. Neural Comput 9(7):1483–1492. https://doi.org/10.1162/neco.1997.9.7.1483

Hyvärinen A, Köster U (2006) FastISA: A fast fixed-point algorithm for independent subspace analysis. In: Proc ESANN 2006, Bruges, Belgium, pp 371–376

Hyvärinen A, Karhunen J, Oja E (2002) Independent component analysis, 1st edn. Wiley, New York, NY

Ioffe S, Szegedy C (2015) Batch normalization: Accelerating deep network training by reducing internal covariate shift. In: Proc ICML 2015, Lille, France, vol 37, pp 448–456

Karahan E, Rojas-López PA, Bringas-Vega ML, Valdés-Hernández PA, Valdés-Sosa PA (2015) Tensor analysis and fusion of multimodal brain images. Proc IEEE 103(9):1531–1559. https://doi.org/10.1109/JPROC.2015.2455028

Kettenring J (1971) Canonical analysis of several sets of variables. Biometrika 58(3):433–451. https://doi.org/10.2307/2334380
Kim T, Eltoft T, Lee TW (2006) Independent vector analysis: An extension of ICA to multivariate components. In: Proc ICA 2006, Springer, Charleston, SC, Lecture Notes in Computer Science, vol 3889, pp 165–172. https://doi.org/10.1007/11679363_21
Krizhevsky A, Sutskever I, Hinton GE (2012) Imagenet classification with deep convolutional neural networks. In: Proc NIPS 2012, pp 1097–1105
Lahat D, Jutten C (2015) Joint independent subspace analysis: A quasi-Newton algorithm. In: Proc LVA/ICA 2015, Springer, Liberec, Czech Republic, Lecture Notes in Computer Science, vol 9237, pp 111–118. https://doi.org/10.1007/978-3-319-22482-4_13
Lahat D, Cardoso J, Messer H (2012) Second-order multidimensional ICA: Performance analysis. IEEE Trans Signal Process 60(9):4598–4610. https://doi.org/10.1109/TSP.2012.2199985
Lahat D, Adalı T, Jutten C (2015) Multimodal data fusion: An overview of methods, challenges, and prospects. Proc IEEE 103(9):1449–1477. https://doi.org/10.1109/JPROC.2015.2460697
Liu J, Pearlson G, Calhoun V, Windemuth A (2007) A novel approach to analyzing fMRI and SNP data via parallel independent component analysis. Proc SPIE 6511:651,113–651,113–11. https://doi.org/10.1117/12.709344
Liu J, Pearlson G, Windemuth A, Ruano G, Perrone-Bizzozero NI, Calhoun VD (2009) Combining fMRI and SNP data to investigate connections between brain function and genetics using parallel ICA. Hum Brain Mapp 30(1):241–255. https://doi.org/10.1002/hbm.20508
Long J, Shelhamer E, Darrell T (2015) Fully convolutional networks for semantic segmentation. In: Proc IEEE CVPR 2015, pp 3431–3440. https://doi.org/10.1109/CVPR.2015.7298965
Lorenzi M, Simpson IJ, Mendelson AF, Vos SB, Cardoso MJ, Modat M, Schott JM, Ourselin S (2016) Multimodal image analysis in Alzheimer's disease via statistical modelling of non-local intensity correlations. Sci Rep 6:22,161. https://doi.org/10.1038/srep22161
Maaten Lvd, Hinton G (2008) Visualizing data using t-SNE. J Mach Learn Res 9(Nov):2579–2605
Martínez-Montes E, Valdés-Sosa PA, Miwakeichi F, Goldman RI, Cohen MS (2004) Concurrent EEG/fMRI analysis by multiway partial least squares. NeuroImage 22(3):1023–1034. https://doi.org/10.1016/j.neuroimage.2004.03.038
Meda S, Narayanan B, Liu J, Perrone-Bizzozero N, Stevens M, Calhoun VD, Glahn D, Shen L, Risacher S, Saykin A, Pearlson G (2012) A large scale multivariate parallel ICA method reveals novel imaging-genetic relationships for Alzheimer's disease in the ADNI cohort. NeuroImage 60(3):1608–1621. https://doi.org/10.1016/j.neuroimage.2011.12.076
Meier T, Wildenberg J, Liu J, Chen J, Calhoun VD, Biswal B, Meyerand M, Birn R, Prabhakaran V (2012) Parallel ICA identifies sub-components of resting state networks that covary with behavioral indices. Front Hum Neurosci 6:281. https://doi.org/10.3389/fnhum.2012.00281
Miller KL, Alfaro-Almagro F, Bangerter NK, Thomas DL, Yacoub E, Xu J, Bartsch AJ, Jbabdi S, Sotiropoulos SN, Andersson JLR, Griffanti L, Douaud G, Okell TW, Weale P, Dragonu I, Garratt S, Hudson S, Collins R, Jenkinson M, Matthews PM, Smith SM (2016) Multimodal population brain imaging in the UK Biobank prospective epidemiological study. Nat Neurosci 19(11):1523–1536. https://doi.org/10.1038/nn.4393
Mohammadi-Nejad AR, Hossein-Zadeh GA, Soltanian-Zadeh H (2017) Structured and sparse canonical correlation analysis as a brain-wide multi-modal data fusion approach. IEEE Trans Med Imaging 36(7):1438–1448. https://doi.org/10.1109/TMI.2017.2681966
Plis SM, Hjelm DR, Salakhutdinov R, Allen EA, Bockholt HJ, Long JD, Johnson HJ, Paulsen JS, Turner JA, Calhoun VD (2014) Deep learning for neuroimaging: a validation study. Front Neurosci 8:229. https://doi.org/10.3389/fnins.2014.00229
Silva RF, Plis SM, Adalı T, Calhoun VD (2014a) Multidataset independent subspace analysis. In: Proc OHBM 2014, Poster 3506
Silva RF, Plis SM, Adalı T, Calhoun VD (2014b) Multidataset independent subspace analysis extends independent vector analysis. In: Proc IEEE ICIP 2014, Paris, France, pp 2864–2868. https://doi.org/10.1109/ICIP.2014.7025579

Silva RF, Plis SM, Adalı T, Calhoun VD (2014c) A statistically motivated framework for simulation of stochastic data fusion models applied to multimodal neuroimaging. NeuroImage 102, Part 1:92–117. https://doi.org/10.1016/j.neuroimage.2014.04.035

Silva RF, Plis SM, Sui J, Pattichis MS, Adalı T, Calhoun VD (2016) Blind source separation for unimodal and multimodal brain networks: A unifying framework for subspace modeling. IEEE J Sel Topics Signal Process 10(7):1134–1149. https://doi.org/10.1109/JSTSP.2016.2594945

Srivastava N, Hinton G, Krizhevsky A, Sutskever I, Salakhutdinov R (2014) Dropout: A simple way to prevent neural networks from overfitting. J Mach Learn Res 15:1929–1958

Sui J, Adalı T, Pearlson G, Yange H, Sponheim S, White T, Calhoun V (2010) A CCA + ICA based model for multi-task brain imaging data fusion and its application to schizophrenia. NeuroImage 51(1):123–134. https://doi.org/10.1016/j.neuroimage.2010.01.069

Sui J, Pearlson G, Caprihan A, Adalı T, Kiehl K, Liu J, Yamamoto J, Calhoun VD (2011) Discriminating schizophrenia and bipolar disorder by fusing fMRI and DTI in a multimodal CCA + joint ICA model. NeuroImage 57(3):839–855. https://doi.org/10.1016/j.neuroimage.2011.05.055

Sui J, He H, Yu Q, Chen J, Rogers J, Pearlson G, Mayer A, Bustillo J, Canive J, Calhoun VD (2013) Combination of resting state fMRI, DTI and sMRI data to discriminate schizophrenia by N-way MCCA+jICA. Front Hum Neurosci 7(235). https://doi.org/10.3389/fnhum.2013.00235

Szabó Z, Póczos B, Lőrincz A (2012) Separation theorem for independent subspace analysis and its consequences. Pattern Recognit 45(4):1782–1791. https://doi.org/10.1016/j.patcog.2011.09.007

Ulloa A, Plis S, Erhardt E, Calhoun V (2015) Synthetic structural magnetic resonance image generator improves deep learning prediction of schizophrenia. In: Proc IEEE MLSP 2015, pp 1–6. https://doi.org/10.1109/MLSP.2015.7324379

Ulloa A, Plis SM, Calhoun VD (2018) Improving classification rate of schizophrenia using a multimodal multi-layer perceptron model with structural and functional MR. arXiv preprint URL http://arxiv.org/abs/1804.04591

Vergara VM, Ulloa A, Calhoun VD, Boutte D, Chen J, Liu J (2014) A three-way parallel ICA approach to analyze links among genetics, brain structure and brain function. NeuroImage 98:386–394. https://doi.org/10.1016/j.neuroimage.2014.04.060

Wang P, Chen K, Yao L, Hu B, Wu X, Zhang J, Ye Q, Guo X (2016) Multimodal classification of mild cognitive impairment based on partial least squares. J Alzheimers Dis 54(1):359–371. https://doi.org/10.3233/JAD-160102

Wold H (1966) Nonlinear estimation by iterative least squares procedures. In: David F (ed) Research papers in statistics. Festschrift for J. Neyman. Wiley, New York, NY, pp 411–444

Yeredor A (2000) Blind separation of gaussian sources via second-order statistics with asymptotically optimal weighting. IEEE Signal Process Lett 7(7):197–200. https://doi.org/10.1109/97.847367

Zhou YT, Chellappa R (1988) Computation of optical flow using a neural network. In: Proc IEEE ICNN 1988, vol 2, pp 71–78. https://doi.org/10.1109/ICNN.1988.23914

Ethics in the Era of Big Data

9

Diego Librenza-Garcia

9.1 Initial Considerations

Technology and its consequences in human behavior and relationships have been fascinating mankind for centuries. A whole new literary genre was created with science fiction so that we could imaginatively explore what the future may hold for our species. Since then, both movies and novels have increasingly focused on technological advancement, == most often in dystopic scenarios, in which artificial intelligence creates prejudice and ethical dilemmas through biased handling of personal and collective data. Despite these catastrophic predictions, technological progress* has redefined our civilization and our way of life with exponential advances, to the point that some publications, such as The Economist, declared that data might be considered for this century what oil was to the last one, conceiving a whole new economic scenario (Economist 2017). In medicine, and more particularly in psychiatry, big data analytics represent a new era in which we are shifting from group-level evidence, as proposed by medicine-based evidence, to individual and personalized predictions, potentially leading to personalized care (Greenhalgh et al. 2014; Passos et al. 2016). Nevertheless, despite all prospects regarding the growth, sharing and processing of data, and all the benefits it may represent, this revolution does not come without risks.

To appear in Ives Passos, Benson Mwangi, and Flávio Kapczinski (Eds.) *Personalized and Predictive Psychiatry - Big Data Analytics in Mental Health*. NY: Springer Nature.

D. Librenza-Garcia (✉)
Department of Psychiatry and Behavioural Neurosciences, McMaster University, Mood Disorders Program, Hamilton, ON, Canada

Graduation Program in Psychiatry and Department of Psychiatry, Federal University of Rio Grande do Sul (UFRGS), Porto Alegre, Brazil
e-mail: librenzagarcia@gmail.com

I. C. Passos et al., *Personalized Psychiatry*,
https://doi.org/10.1007/978-3-030-03553-2_9

Although data, per se, is ethically neutral, what one decides to do with it may not be. Estimates point that in 2018, 50% of business ethics violations may happen through improper handling of these large data sets and its analysis (Herschel and Miori 2017). As most revolutions go, we are noticing both the benefits and the problems related to Big Data as it unfolds, and most of the time, by seeing its negative consequences and reacting to them rather than acting proactively.* However there is an optimistic* view of how big data and techniques such as machine learning may improve health services in all respects. (Barrett et al. 2013; Angus 2015; Insel and Cuthbert 2015; Huys et al. 2016; Beam and Kohane 2018). Not only can this* improve hospital and doctor performance, but also an individual's quality of life and how patients understand and interact with these disorders (or the perspective of presenting them in the future). On the other hand, we are unaware of how big data may negatively impact* these same dimensions or create new types of inequality.

The present chapter provides a perspective on the ethical issues that may emerge from big data analytics and how this may challenge us in the coming years. Although ethics may have many definitions that go than "what is right and what is wrong," an ongoing field must adapt to new realities as well as the ethical issues and the discussion of how to deal with them may have many definitions that go well beyond "what is right and what is wrong"'* paramount (Davis 2012). In fact, we are already experiencing the impact of big data for many years now and may see its influence exponentially increasing in the next years. For this chapter, we chose to divide the ethical challenges into four sections. First, regarding the data itself and its handling. Second, the impact that predictive models created with this data may have for patients. Third, the ethical issues created by these same models to clinicians, and fourth, the ethical issues involved in research, especially regarding informed consent.

9.2 Ethical Issues Regarding Data

Data has been created since the beginning of civilization, first in the form of pictures drawn by our ancestors in caves, then by written registers and, nowadays, created, stored and processed by a myriad of electronic devices that are continually registering and creating information (World Economic Forum 2011; Lantz 2015; Beam and Kohane 2018). What changed recently is the speed at which we create and store data and the fact that now we have both the methods and the computational capacity to extract useful insights from this vast amount of information (Lantz 2015). However, from the collecting to the application of this massive flow of data, some questions arise. Who owns this information, and how can it be used? How may this constant flow harm individual privacy, or how may a lack of transparency facilitate a data monopoly, where a minority of individuals may consolidate power and control? of transparency generate. The legislation is still emerging and many of these questions remain open to discussion, and we are probably looking at two opposing risks. First, that data may be poorly handled and create negative consequences for individual and society; and second, that the perception of this threat may lead to disproportional overregulation that could slow down and delay the positive effects of big data.

9.2.1 Privacy and Anonymity

It is hard to think of any human activity nowadays that does not generate data, given how connected we are with electronic devices and, in consequence, interconnected with each other. Our behavior produces a data imprint, which may allow others to detect our behavioral patterns, and reveal our personal preferences* (Davis 2012; Murdoch and Detsky 2013). Although terms of service from software that collect personal data usually mention privacy and assure data anonymity, they can sometimes be vague and superficial in their description. In some cases, one can analyze this "anonymized data" and through reverse engineering, trace information back to a singular individual, a process called re-identification (Tene and Polonetsky 2013; Mello et al. 2013; Terry 2014). This precedent is of extreme importance in the medical setting, as health-related data may contain sensitive information about the patients, such as sexual orientation, previous history of abortions, suicide attempts and so on. Moreover, patients are vulnerable because of their expectations regarding their diagnosis or apprehension towards treatment and prognosis, and the disclosure of this information may complicate even more how they experience their disorder or treatment.

It is also essential to determine who should have access to data and for what purpose. Re-identification or hackings may lead to data leakage and exposure of sensitive information, but physical and remote access to stored data may also give an individual opportunity of duplicating a data set and releasing this information (Culnan and Williams 2009). Those who are granted direct access* to the data and handle it in their daily work are in a position of power. Companies and institutions need to establish clear policies to determine who is granted access to this information, to avoid sensitive data to be inadequately visualized, analyzed and exposed (Davis 2012).

Given how dynamic Big Data is, it is almost impossible to actively monitor how private information is being stored and propagated. Agreement terms that indicate that data will be used to "personalize experience" or "improve performance" may fail to inform, for example, if that data is being sold or transferred to third parties—a widespread practice—and for what those third parties may use it. The same information may have very different uses: one can create models based on social media information for very different tasks, such as selling a product or predicting harmful behavior such as suicide attempt. When an individual agrees to share their data, how exactly and for what these data is used are questions that either remain unanswered or are answered without the pertinent specificity. In the particular case of social media, although information is in a public virtual space, people may be unaware of its multiple uses and the commercial value of what they are producing. Lastly, there is a risk that anonymized data may be clustered according to geographical, ethnic or last sexual orientation, that may lead to discrimination and stigmatization—in this case, affecting not only the individuals that share their data but also others in these clusters (Craig and Ludloff 2011; Schadt 2012; Mittelstadt and Floridi 2016).

9.2.2 Ownership

Since we are unceasingly producing data, which is continuously being stored, who does this data belong to exactly? It is unthinkable that all this information can be managed by the individual that generates it across the unending stream of information that goes from our devices to corporations and governments, and then back to the individual in the form of actions or products. How much value can be assigned to a given amount of information, and can a corporation sell a given individual's personal data? It is somewhat disturbing that someone might own people's personal information, as well as their behavior and preferences, and may employ these to influence future behavior and preferences. The boundaries here are also uncertain: which data may be public and which data may remain private? Which data may lie in between, accessible for purposes of research and innovation but not entirely public? From the moment a patient enters an emergency room until its discharge several days later, he generates a variety of data. Should the institution be free to use all kinds of data, some of them, or none, and whom may have access to the raw data and the insights extracted from it? It is unarguable how useful this information is, but there are no universal regulations on the matter. Furthermore, ownership may be defined not by only possessing the rights to compile and use with exclusivity the data, but also to the right of analyzing and use it to create new technologies, generating copyrighted products or patents (Choudhury et al. 2014).

9.2.3 Transparency

Data gathering services should not only be transparent about what they are collecting and what are the potential uses of the data, but they should state this in a clear and concise way. A study found that, if one stops to read each term of agreement in a year, one would waste approximately 76 work days reading them (McDonald and Cranor 2008). When an individual is sharing his data, it is relevant to know the ethical principles of the institution in charge of the data gathering, what they intend to do with the information and what is out of boundaries (Davis 2012; Liyanage et al. 2014). In recent years, we have seen many cases in which data was secretly collected and analyzed, and with no purpose known to the users of the service (van der Sloot 2015). Despite the violation of the individual autonomy, this course of action may discourage people from sharing their data even in reliable and transparent platforms, thus limiting the data available for analysis. As already pointed out, it should be clear if the data set would be shared with third parties, or sold to them, or even aggregate external sources.

9.2.4 Identity and Reputation

Technological advancements have altered the way we see ourselves as individuals. Nowadays, our identity consists of both our offline and online activities, and our reputation is influenced by our behavior in both these dimensions. Our offline behavior may impact our online reputation and vice-versa (Davis 2012; Andrejevic 2014). In this sense, the possibility of sensitive data exposure as a result of re-identification or hacking may have an impact in the offline and online parts of people's identity, and therefore harming their reputation. It is not clear how some platforms deal with sensitive in some cases and how much it is protected. Even if agencies with highly classified information are hacked, it is worrisome to think how vulnerable other information may be, such as electronic records or private files. A breach of privacy, therefore, may lead to irreversible and harmful repercussions in how we and others perceive ourselves.

9.2.5 Reliability

Beyond the traditional "3 V's" of Big Data—Variety, Velocity, Volume—IBM proposed a fourth V, veracity (Zikopoulos et al. 2012). Data is not always reliable—it could be human error or bias when a person is collecting the data, or perhaps the use of an uncalibrated device that gives wrong measures, or just the fact that subjects of interest may opt-out, with loss of relevant information. The analysis of incomplete, biased or out of context data may lead to incorrect conclusions, and those conclusions may lead to harmful action or decisions (Bail 2014; Markowetz et al. 2014). Moreover, data is increasingly becoming collected autonomously, by sensor devices, and not infrequently, being processed and analyzed independently of human interference also. The complexity of algorithms used in this analysis—the so called black box methods—may result in our inability to understand how they work, which is troublesome when these same algorithms may be used to influence behavior or make decisions with high impact on one's treatment and prognosis, for example (Lantz 2015).

We should avoid models that are biased in nature. For example, when creating an algorithm to predict suicide attempts, via collecting social media data, users may not be representative of those who use another platform, or those who, although have an account, are not active. Although it may be argued that not being active is also valuable information, this model will fail to identify suicide attempts among inactive individuals of this network, that may be generating relevant data in another platform that is relevant to the topic of interest. On the other hand, a universal model including all internet-related information plus offline use of devices for the individual may be closer to the aim of predicting suicide—although with higher costs and astounding complexity. Before applying any algorithm in real life scenarios, we should take these problems into account, to prevent that biased models with incorrect or incomplete conclusions ended up causing more harm than benefit (Andrejevic 2014).

9.3 Ethical Issues Regarding Patients

Predictive psychiatry may contribute to improve outcomes and prevent disability or harm, but it may also produce harm, influencing other spheres beyond individual's health. If we can predict that an individual will have a more pernicious illness course, that would mean he will make more use of health services, and therefore, may be charged more for a health plan. The prediction, per se, may not be an issue, but the application may perhaps be. For instance, it may be possible that unfavourable outcomes of an individual may fuel eugenic policies or even create social prejudice regarding the subjects with these outcomes.

We should also worry about how devastating a prediction could be. One classic example is Huntington's disease, an autosomal dominant disorder that can be predicted by a simple genetic test. A positive test may tell a patient that he will, in the next years, experience a progressive and severe loss of its brain functions, while the subject is still healthy. If an individual is predicted to develop a psychiatric disorder years before its onset, how many this information influence his quality of life, or ability to avoid that outcome? How will it influence his relationships with his peers or change the course of his actions in the scenario where he was not informed of the outcome? It is possible that the stressful burden of knowing may incur in speeding the disorder installment or even lead to another disorder, such as a depressive episode or substance abuse, in the prior years before the onset of the predicted disorder. A question of the uttermost importance in big data ethics is how our patients may cope with such predictions about their future, and weigh harm and benefit of its use. It is different if we develop an intervention to prevent the outcome and can offer it to an individual. The following clinical cases illustrate some of these ethical dilemmas.

Case 1

J. is an 18-year old male who decides to enlist and serve in the Army. After collecting a series of clinical data and undergo neuroimage acquisition and analysis of serum biomarkers, he is predicted to develop PTSD along with a mood disorder during his time serving with 98% accuracy. Moreover, the algorithm also predicted with an accuracy of 92% that he would attempt suicide in the following year. He still wants to serve the Army even knowing the risks. However, he is then dismissed against his will.

Case 2
C. is a 15-year old female whose father has bipolar disorder with a pernicious trajectory marked by functional impairment and disability, as well as metabolic disorders. At the will of her mother, she underwent a test that can predict with almost 100% accuracy if one will develop a psychiatric disorder in the future. She is then predicted to develop bipolar disorder with a similar course of her father in the next ten years. There is no available treatment at the time to prevent this conversion.

Although big data analytics may have several benefits and a substantial social impact to prevent outcomes such as PTSD, one may argue that there is no absolute prediction and that the individual may have the autonomy to choose to serve the army regardless. However, from a legal perspective, enlist an individual with high chances of developing a debilitating disorder may incur in health-care related expenses and pensions. Moreover, if he develops a disorder on the battlefield, it is possible that his symptoms may jeopardize his safety and that of other soldiers. There is also a possibility of joining the Army but not be sent to the field—which may stigmatize J. as being unable for some medical reason to go to combat.

In the second scenario, knowing that C. will most likely develop BD may help in screening her for the first symptoms of the disorder and allow early intervention when needed. She may start attending an outpatient clinic before the installment of the disorder. She will probably need familiar and professionalized support throughout this prodromal period. Again, there is a chance she will not develop the disorder cause the prediction is not perfectly accurate, and she may undergo all this traumatic experience unnecessarily. Also, as she is a minor, should her mother decide she does not need to know at this point, what course of action should the psychiatrist take?

What is common to both cases is the uncertainty of the prediction. It is hard to imagine a 100% accurate application to predict an outcome, at least with our current state-of-the-art resources. There is always the possibility of that outcome not happening, and the individual forced to live with the burden of its possibility. Although most algorithms and models in current studies are still in proof-of-concept phases so far, it is possible that patients should experience this dilemma in the future. In this uncharted territory, there is no delimited policy or guidelines on how to proceed, nor protocols available for follow-up and assessment. Medical guidelines may have to address the problem of "potential patients," that do not manifest any symptoms at the time of the prediction.

9.4 Ethical Issues Regarding Clinician Decision

We can hypothesize at some point in the future, machines may provide diagnoses with better accuracy than physicians, as some algorithms are already achieving higher accuracies with machine learning than doctors to diagnose certain conditions

(Liu et al. 2017). They can also be used to redefine diagnosis by grouping patients with similar characteristics and integrating different levels of information in such a convoluted way that the meaning of this categories may be impossible for us to understand (Insel and Cuthbert 2015; Huys et al. 2016). The positive implications include predicting treatment response or detecting a disorder* before its onset and may alert us which patients will experience unfavorable functional or cognitive outcomes and have a more severe illness course (Passos et al. 2016; Librenza-Garcia et al. 2017). Predictive models open a door not only to prevention of these outcomes due to early intervention strategies but also to efforts to avoid conversion to a disorder. Amidst all these advances, the clinician finds himself as a bridge between patient and machine, trying to deal with patient expectations and technological insights.

Technology, however, is still dependent on our input. We have to define a psychiatric disorder and the outcome for the machine to interpret, and if we do it wrong, all data and inferences about it would be, in consequence, useless. Machines could get insight on data that we cannot, but we still need to interpret its findings. We can data mine for clusters of patients and redefine the way we diagnose, but given the number of different ways this could go, we should still choose which road we will take from there. At least in psychiatry, it is unimaginable—for now—to think that a machine could replace the clinician, given the importance of empathy and the doctor-patient relationship. The two cases below illustrate some challenges in clinician decision.

Case 3

A psychiatrist will discharge an inpatient after a month of hospitalization. He performs a standard battery of exams and gather clinical data and uses a phone application that can predict suicide attempt in the next three months with high accuracy. Despite being euthymic and with no suicidal ideation at the time, the patient is predicted to attempt suicide in this period.

Case 4

After a series of appointments in an outpatient clinic, the psychiatrist evaluating F. gives him a diagnosis of major depressive disorder. By gathering genetic, neuroimaging, clinical and serum biomarkers data, an algorithm predicts with a high accuracy that the patient has, in fact, bipolar disorder. The psychiatrist, then, reconsiders his choice of monotherapy with an antidepressant.

It is very likely that predictions may impact on clinician decision. If the patient in case 3 is predicted to attempt suicide, should he stay in inpatient care for a greater amount of time, or go home with familiar surveillance and regular appointments? If he lives alone, should he receive domiciliary follow-up as well? If by one side this prediction may provide better resource assignments for those predicted to attempt suicide, it can also lead to neglection of those predicted not to undergo this outcome. Since no model is perfect, some of the high-risk individuals may receive a regular follow-up, and the clinician may relax and neglect important risk signs, reassured by the negative prediction. In the case of F., despite the clinical diagnosis, the psychiatry may be reluctant cause the depressive episode may be only a first manifestation of bipolar disorder and may be followed by a manic presentation in the future—in the worst-case scenario, an iatrogenic manic switch triggered by his choice of treatment. On the other hand, if the prediction is wrong, he may be depriving the patient of a first line treatment and using an additional and unnecessary mood stabilizer, with all its known side effects.

9.5 Ethical Issues in Research

Informed consents in psychiatric research are usually developed stating what data will be collected and to what end. This poses a challenge because one of the purposes of big data analytics is to extract new knowledge or patterns from that information, ones that may not be included in the initial aim of a study—especially if we are dealing with unsupervised models. So, it is a challenge on how to include the unpredictable in the informed consent. Patients usually consent to participate in a single study, but big data may be more useful if data is shared, integrated and reanalyzed between different groups, increasing its complexity but also providing us with even more useful insights (Ioannidis 2013; Larson 2013; Choudhury et al. 2014). Also, we usually do not state for patients if whatever insight we obtained from the data may result in any feedback to them. If we create a model to predict response to antidepressants that have high accuracy and applicability, and it predicts that a patient in the validate sample will relapse with the medication he is currently using, will he be informed? Although this sound logical, should we also inform a patient if the accuracy is relevant, but not applicable?

Another relevant question is how we should handle social media information. Although it may have been made public, is the individual aware that his information can be used in a health-related scenario? How should we gather consent in such a vast universe? (Krotoski 2012; Lomborg and Bechmann 2014). One may hypothesize that in the future an individual may "opt-in" to data in which he is willing to share, and for which application*, but for now, each platform, software or website has a different policy (Prainsack and Buyx 2013). Broader consent policy may resolve the issue on the end of big data but not of the individual while listing possible future uses and authorization for each may be more comfortable for the patient but limit newer insights into that data in the future. Reassessment for new consent can also be one strategy, but it will probably reduce the sample due to follow-up losses (Currie 2013; Lomborg and Bechmann 2014). Moreover, it would increase the costs and bureaucracy and slow down or preclude future research.

The fact is, for most of our studies, informed consent was designed to tackle themes relevant to evidence-based medicine, with predefined questions and a limited amount of answers expected. From now on, it is necessary to find a way to adapt it to this new reality, which includes the uncertainty of what the data can reveal and how it can impact patients afterward.

9.6 Conclusion

In the past, we would not dare to dream how big data would defy our limits and see far beyond what we can, nor how it could expand the limits of the world by not only redefining the real world but also creating uncountable virtual ones. It is undeniable that Big data is pushing us to consider ethical issues and whether they violate fundamental, civil, social, political or legal rights. On the other hand, big data analytics will also redefine what we think is possible in the next few years, with the possibility of devices being even more ingrained in our daily patterns of behavior, through digital profiling, and artificially intelligent-driven politics. The aforementioned ethical issues are only the ones we are facing now and in the near future. New issues may arise in areas that do not even exist at this time, and more challenges will surface as big data technology continues to evolve and expand its influence in our lives. There is no telling how much we will advance and how far the possibilities of this evolution may lead us, and what unforeseen ethical issues may arise ahead. Whether big data and artificial intelligence will guide us towards a dystopic or utopic society, it depends on how we will handle these ethical issues from now on. Technology, like every resource, is primarily neutral and can be used to cause both benefit and harm.

There is a delicate balance that we shall seek for the sake of an efficient and human health-care. A lack of policies on how to handle and utilize data may result in more inequality and create unpredictable harm to society and individuals. Nevertheless, if society lets itself to be driven by unfounded concerns about these new technologies, it may overreact and create preemptive obstacles, to the point in which a restrictive and overregulated policy may prevent not only harm but also progress and benefits that could improve patient care and change illness' course.

Some of the values we have today may evolve as new challenges arrive, which will promote a reformulation of our ethical principles. In this fashion, big data ethics do not consist of absolute and immutable principles, but, on the opposite, it is malleable according to the challenges and outcomes not prior anticipated. Some scenarios presented in this chapter are already challenging, and there is no telling what new ones may lie ahead. Nevertheless, besides all potential innovations and problematic scenarios big data may cause, one fundamental principle of medicine stated in the Hippocratic Oath still applies: *primum non nocere (First, to do no harm).*

Acknowledgement and Disclaimer The author has no conflicts of interest.

References

Andrejevic M (2014) The big data divide. Int J Commun 8:1673–1689. 1932–8036/20140005

Angus DC (2015) (NIG) fusing randomized trials with big data: the key to self-learning health care systems? JAMA J Am Med Assoc 314:767–768. https://doi.org/10.1001/jama.2015.7762

Bail CA (2014) The cultural environment: measuring culture with big data. Theory Soc 43:465–524. https://doi.org/10.1007/s11186-014-9216-5

Barrett MA, Humblet O, Hiatt RA, Adler NE (2013) Big data and disease prevention: *from quantified self to quantified communities*. Big Data 1:168–175. https://doi.org/10.1089/big.2013.0027

Beam AL, Kohane IS (2018) Big data and machine learning in health care. JAMA J Am Med Assoc 319:1317–1318. https://doi.org/10.1001/jama.2017.18391

Choudhury S, Fishman JR, McGowan ML, Juengst ET (2014) Big data, open science and the brain: lessons learned from genomics. Front Hum Neurosci 8:1–10. https://doi.org/10.3389/fnhum.2014.00239

Craig T, Ludloff ME (2011) Privacy and big data: the players, regulators, and stakeholders. O'Reilly Media

Culnan MJ, Williams CC (2009) How ethics can enhance organizational privacy: lessons from the choicepoint and TJX data breaches. MIS Q 33:673–687. https://doi.org/10.2307/20650322

Currie J (2013) "Big data" versus "big brother": on the appropriate use of large-scale data collections in pediatrics. Pediatrics 131:S127–S132. https://doi.org/10.1542/peds.2013-0252c

Davis K (2012) Ethics of big data: balancing risk and innovation. O'Reilly Media

Economist T (2017) The world's most valuable resource is no longer oil, but data. Econ

Greenhalgh T, Howick J, Maskrey N (2014) Evidence based medicine: a movement in crisis. BMJ 348:g3725–g3725. https://doi.org/10.1136/bmj.g3725

Herschel R, Miori VM (2017) Ethics & big data. Technol Soc 49:31–36. https://doi.org/10.1016/j.techsoc.2017.03.003

Huys QJM, Maia TV, Frank MJ (2016) Computational psychiatry as a bridge from neuroscience to clinical applications. Nat Neurosci 19:404–413. https://doi.org/10.1038/nn.4238

Insel TR, Cuthbert BN (2015) Brain disorders? Precisely. Science 348:499–500. https://doi.org/10.1126/science.aab2358

Ioannidis JPA (2013) Informed consent, big data, and the oxymoron of research that is not research. Am J Bioeth 13:40–42. https://doi.org/10.1080/15265161.2013.768864

Krotoski AK (2012) Data-driven research: open data opportunities for growing knowledge, and ethical issues that arise. Insights UKSG J 25:28–32. https://doi.org/10.1629/2048-7754.25.1.28

Lantz B (2015) Machine learning with R - second edition. Cambridge University Press, Cambridge

Larson EB (2013) Building trust in the power of "big data" research to serve the public good. JAMA 309:2443. https://doi.org/10.1001/jama.2013.5914

Librenza-Garcia D, Kotzian BJ, Yang J et al (2017) The impact of machine learning techniques in the study of bipolar disorder: a systematic review. Neurosci Biobehav Rev 80:538–554. https://doi.org/10.1016/j.neubiorev.2017.07.004

Liu Y, Gadepalli K, Norouzi M, et al (2017) Detecting cancer metastases on gigapixel pathology images. 1–13. https://doi.org/10.1016/j.ejim.2017.06.017

Liyanage H, De Lusignan S, Liaw S et al (2014) Big data usage patterns in the health care domain: a use case driven approach applied to the assessment of vaccination benefits and risks contribution of the IMIA primary healthcare working group big data for assessing vaccination benefits and risks: A. IMIA. Yearb Med Inform:27–35

Lomborg S, Bechmann A (2014) Using APIs for data collection on social media. Inf Soc 30:256–265. https://doi.org/10.1080/01972243.2014.915276

Markowetz A, Błaszkiewicz K, Montag C et al (2014) Psycho-informatics: big data shaping modern psychometrics. Med Hypotheses 82:405–411. https://doi.org/10.1016/j.mehy.2013.11.030

McDonald AM, Cranor LF (2008) The cost of reading privacy policies. A J Law Policy Inf Soc 4:543–568

Mello MM, Francer JK, Wilenzick M et al (2013) Preparing for responsible sharing of clinical trial data. N Engl J Med 369:1651–1658. https://doi.org/10.1056/NEJMhle1309073

Mittelstadt BD, Floridi L (2016) The ethics of big data: current and foreseeable issues in biomedical contexts. Sci Eng Ethics 22:303–341. https://doi.org/10.1007/s11948-015-9652-2

Murdoch TBTB, Detsky ASAS (2013) The inevitable application of big data to health care. JAMA 309:1351–1352. https://doi.org/10.1001/jama.2013.393

Passos IC, Mwangi B, Kapczinski F (2016) Big data analytics and machine learning: 2015 and beyond. Lancet Psychiatry 3:13–15. https://doi.org/10.1016/S2215-0366(15)00549-0

Prainsack B, Buyx A (2013) A solidarity-based approach to the governance of research biobanks. Med Law Rev 21:71–91. https://doi.org/10.1093/medlaw/fws040

Schadt EE (2012) The changing privacy landscape in the era of big data. Mol Syst Biol 8:1–3. https://doi.org/10.1038/msb.2012.47

Tene O, Polonetsky J (2013) Big data for all: privacy and user control in the age of analytics

Terry N (2014) Health privacy is difficult but not impossible in a post-HIPAA data-driven world. Chest 146:835–840. https://doi.org/10.1378/chest.13-2909

van der Sloot B (2015) How to assess privacy violations in the age of big data? Analysing the three different tests developed by the ECtHR and adding for a fourth one. Inf Commun Technol Law 24:74–103. https://doi.org/10.1080/13600834.2015.1009714

World Economic Forum (2011) Personal data: the emergence of a new asset class

Zikopoulos PC, DeRoos D, Parasuraman K, et al (2012) Harness the power of big data

Index

I. C. Passos et al., *Personalized Psychiatry*,
https://doi.org/10.1007/978-3-030-03553-2

MIX
Papier aus verantwortungsvollen Quellen
Paper from responsible sources
FSC® C105338
FSC
www.fsc.org

If you have any concerns about our products,
you can contact us on
ProductSafety@springernature.com

In case Publisher is established outside the EU,
the EU authorized representative is:
Springer Nature Customer Service Center GmbH
Europaplatz 3, 69115 Heidelberg, Germany

Printed by Libri Plureos GmbH
in Hamburg, Germany